Clinics in Developmental Medicine No. 75

A Neurophysiological Basis
for the
Treatment of Cerebral Palsy

2nd Edition of CDM 23
*The Motor Deficit in Patients
with Cerebral Palsy*

By

KAREL BOBATH

Preface by

Martin C. O. Bax

1980

Spastics International Medical Publications

LONDON: William Heinemann Medical Books Ltd.

PHILADELPHIA: J. B. Lippincott Co.

ISBN 0433 03335 5

Printed in England at THE LAVENHAM PRESS LTD., Lavenham, Suffolk

Contents

Preface to Second Edition

The first edition of this book has proved to be one of the most popular of the *Clinics in Developmental Medicine*. Apart from the personal charisma of the author and his wife Berta, who have linked this theoretical account of their work to their very personal teaching all over the world, there are other reasons why this book has proved popular with doctors and therapists alike.

Despite the strides that have been made in neurophysiological work in recent years much of the work, concentrating perhaps on single cell studies, has not contributed anything new to our understanding of the basis of control of movement or of the nature of motor disorders. Here Karel Bobath's extensive knowledge of the work of the older generation of neurophysiologists stands him (and us) in good stead. No clearer account of some of the underlying motor patterns and responses exists.

In revising the book Dr. Bobath, apart from bringing the work up to date, has sought to clarify his account of motor development and hence this new edition will, I believe, prove even more popular than the previous one. All those interested in motor development and motor handicap will want it on their bookshelves.

Martin C. O. Bax

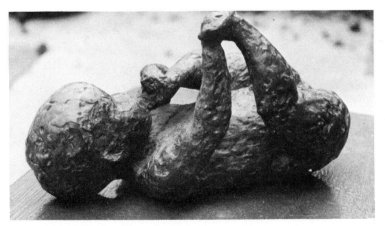

B.B.

Acknowledgements

This small book is the result of dealing with the problems of over 35 years work in the field of cerebral palsy and allied conditions. It reflects the background of treatment along neurological lines, an approach which has been evolved gradually. While the book is not directly concerned with treatment, it gives its background and tries to describe the basic concept underlying treatment. I am conscious of the fact that the concept presented is largely speculative; indeed, it can only be hypothetical and leaves many problems of treatment and management unanswered. During all these years, the treatment has not been methodical, it has not been in any way rigid, but has constantly been developed and changed as observation and experience grew.

I wish to thank all my friends, doctors and therapists, all over the world, who by their criticism and exchange of experience have helped in the perfection of the concept. I want especially to express my profound gratitude to my wife, who by empirically developing the treatment and by constant observation and modification of it has challenged me, kept me from getting rusty and, above all, helped me to fulfil my life's ambition, to learn and to teach. (Where I say 'we' in text, I am in fact referring to my wife and myself). My thanks are due also to the editorial staff of S.I.M.P.

Preface to First Edition

Recent years have seen an increasing interest taken in cerebral palsy as well as in other previously neglected chronic illnesses of childhood. The associated increased interest in the whole field of neurological and psychological disorders of childhood has led to closer study of earlier stages of development. Simultaneously paediatrics has advanced into the study of the newborn and of his neurology. These changes and the special interest of paediatrics in prevention are leading to earlier diagnosis and treatment.

To our better understanding of the underlying neuropathophysiology and treatment of cerebral palsy Karel and Berta Bobath have, I believe, made a great contribution, probably the major contribution.

The learning of voluntary movement appears to depend on the achievement of the movement. More fundamentally it is based on the sensation of the movement. This applies in the normal child's learning and in that of the child with a motor handicap. Treatment by physiotherapy includes active and passive movement but only active movement can give the sensations essential for the learning of voluntary movement.

If the motor education of the child with cerebral palsy is postponed to an age at which he can cooperate actively, treatment will be neglected during the earlier years, and he will have, by the time he can participate in his treatment, acquired many disordered patterns. Yet passive movement cannot teach willed movement.

By using the automatic postural responses present from an early age, the Bobaths solved this apparently insoluble problem. The child who is too young to cooperate can still be induced to make active movements. In addition the development of disadvantageous patterns and postures can be diminished, for the Bobaths have shown that much of the disordered posture and movement typical of cerebral palsy are the result of unchecked postural responses either persisting to abnormally late age or abnormal in other ways.

The more recent application of their ideas in the very early treatment of infants under the age of one year, before the disordered postures and movements are established, suggests that in many cases much of the disorder may be prevented—a most exciting possibility.

The validity of treatment methods in cerebral palsy is not easy to establish. But it is at least more inviting to undertake research on methods which appear to have a sound neurophysiological basis.

In this book Dr. Karel Bobath sets out the neurophysiological mechanisms which underlie the motor disorders of cerebral palsy. They also form the logical basis of the techniques of treatment which Mrs. Berta Bobath and he have advocated and which have won world-wide acceptance.

Their teaching has had great influence for good for they have continuously searched for explanation as well as for better techniques. We are happy to be publishing this book which we believe will be of great usefulness to paediatricians, neurologists, and therapists.

R. C. Mac Keith

CHAPTER 1

Introduction

This analysis of the nature of handicap in children with cerebral palsy is the result of observation and treatment of such children for more than 30 years. The physiological concepts here described serve as a basis for the tests we use, and as a means for diagnosis. They have also guided us in planning treatment and explaining its rationale. While the increased interest in, and knowledge of, the problems of this condition in recent years have resulted in great improvements in diagnosis and early recognition, there is still a large gap between the examination techniques of a paediatric neurologist and the assessment made by therapists for the purpose of planning treatment. They frequently seem to speak a different language and this lack of mutual understanding may be of great disadvantage to the child.

The concept developed here aims to bridge this gap, besides giving the physician a further tool for diagnosis and evaluation, enabling him to predict the further development of the condition, evaluate the response of the child and predict the possibilities of treatment. This is a necessity if the treatment and management of these children is to be successful.

Definition of cerebral palsy

Cerebral palsy is defined as 'a disorder of movement and posture due to a defect or lesion of the immature brain' (Bax 1964). The brain lesion is non-progressive and causes variable impairment of the co-ordination of muscle action, with resulting inability of the child to maintain normal postures and perform normal movements. This central motor handicap is frequently associated with affected speech, vision and hearing, with various types of perceptual disturbances, some degree of mental retardation, and/or epilepsy.

The essential feature of this definition of cerebral palsy is that the lesion affects the immature brain and interferes with the maturation of the CNS, which has specific consequences in terms of the type of cerebral palsy which develops, its diagnosis, assessment and treatment.

Development

A normal baby's development in its totality (physical, mental, emotional and social) depends on his ability to move. Even *in utero* the baby not only sucks his thumb but also presses against the uterine wall and other parts of his own body when moving his limbs, giving him tactile and proprioceptive feedback. From birth the baby continues to touch and explore his body; his fingers go into his mouth; later, his toes and hands come into contact, intertwining. Studies by Kravitz *et al.* (1978) have shown that the baby's exploration of parts of the body by touch is age-related. First he touches his mouth and brings his hands together over his chest, and only later touches

1

more distal parts of his body: for instance, feet and toes around the sixth or seventh month. In this way, by touching his body and by moving, by realising that he can move his hands into the field of vision, the baby develops a body percept during the first 18 months, a feeling of himself as an entity separate from his environment, a knowledge of himself based on visual, tactile and proprioceptive sensations. This will be superseded only much later by the development of a body 'image' with a more visual bias. Once this body percept is established, the infant can begin to relate himself to the world around him and can develop spatial orientation.

A baby deprived by immobility or difficulty in moving and exploring his body, or who can move only in a distorted way, will have difficulty in developing a body percept, or may only do so with difficulty and after a long delay. It is not surprising, therefore, that many of these children may have perceptual difficulties and may appear to be mentally retarded.

Thus it is often difficult to decide whether a child with cerebral palsy suffers from primary or secondary retardation, due to lack of experience caused by his enforced immobility. In our experience, perceptual impairment in these children, especially if discovered early, need not carry the poor prognosis it does in adult life (for instance, in an adult hemiplegic of long standing). In the adult, perceptual disturbances signify damage to specific areas of the central nervous system, or at least interferences with the areas of the brain which subserve some specific perceptual function, whereas in the child with cerebral palsy they do not seem to have localised value, but more often indicate lack of experience or delayed maturation.

The possible delay or arrest in development of these children may also be accentuated by the abnormal development of the mother-child relationship, which is such an important factor in the baby's maturational process. A baby does not mature in a vacuum, he interacts with his environment, especially with his mother, and it seems that some of the early abilities of the baby are especially attuned to establish a strong emotional bond between mother and baby. The cries of a baby are its main language and they have a very strong emotional appeal. Finnish and Swedish doctors (Wasz-Höckert *et al.* 1968) recorded the various types of crying of a number of babies between the ages of 0 to nine months. They recorded the birth cry, the hunger, pain and pleasure cries, and also some typical cries of abnormal babies. The tapes were played back to a group of midwives, doctors and mothers. In a high percentage of cases they were able to interpret the nature of the crying correctly and the mothers were able to pick out their own babies. The emotional appeal of the babies' cries could also often be identified when the recording of the various types of crying was played to a group of students.

A normal baby has a very wide range of behaviour with which to express his needs, likes and dislikes, other than by crying. For example, he can refuse the breast or bottle by turning his head away, he can spit out food he dislikes, he is able to find the nipple or the teat by the rooting reaction when the area round his mouth is touched. *(See footnote on facing page.) Early on he smiles and develops other facial expressions such as frowning and raising his eyebrows. In these and many other ways he establishes a relationship of give-and-take, or interaction between mother and child. Recent studies of at-risk and premature babies

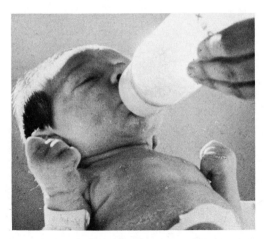

Fig. 1. Normal newborn baby showing close association of sucking reflex and grasp response.

bear out this point. Brimblecombe *et al.* (1978) have stressed the great importance of the early handling of the baby and bodily contact between mother and child for the establishment of a good relationship. It has also been shown how important is the early automatic babbling of the baby in furthering the bond between mother and child. This automatic babbling during the first three months is then sustained by the evoked response from the mother, and is later on transformed into meaningful speech. If babbling stops at about three months it should arouse suspicion of a possible impairment in the baby's hearing.

It seems, therefore, illogical to look upon the various aspects of the baby's development as separate entities. A lesion to the brain, causing cerebral palsy, will interfere to a varying degree with all the aspects of a baby's development. To prevent this seems to be the main argument for the early recognition and management of the condition.

Management

To speak of 'treatment' in this connection is somewhat misleading. 'Management' seems a better term as it indicates not only dealing with the motor handicap, but also with the totality of the child's needs and especially with the establishment of a good mother-child relationship. The main argument for the early recognition and management, of which good physiotherapy is the most important single aspect, is the combination of therapy with a programme of thorough parent training. The establishment of a good mother-child relationship, giving the mother a thorough understanding of the nature of the child's handicap, explaining to her why her child

*If any part of the circumoral area of the baby is touched, he will turn his head until the centre of his mouth engages with the object; this is the rooting reaction, frequently associated with fisting of the hands once the baby begins to suck (Fig. 1). The close association of the rooting and sucking reactions with the grasp response (mentioned by Prechtl 1953) is of great interest. In all animals in early infancy the mouth is the organ of exploration. Only in the ape and man is the function gradually transferred to the arm and hand. This close association explains the not infrequent fact that improvement of grasp and release of the hand in a spastic patient results in improvement of speech and articulation.

3

cannot do certain things, training her in the daily handling of her baby in support of treatment, is far more important than the reasons usually given for early treatment, essential as they are. (It is true, however, that the infantile and immature brain shows much greater plasticity (Gooddy and MacKissock 1951) so that the acquisition and habituation of abnormal patterns of hypertonus could be prevented, and the development of contractures and deformities avoided, thus obviating the need for future corrective surgery—or at least keeping it to distal parts.)

The early recognition of cerebral palsy in its many forms and its differentiation from simple retardation of the development of motor behaviour and from hereditary and congenital conditions, requires a thorough knowledge of the development of motor co-ordination. It is not enough merely to know the usual milestones of motor development as described by Bühler (1927, 1935), Gesell (1940), Gesell and Amatruda (1945, 1947), Griffiths (1954), Illingworth (1960), Hellbrügge and Pechstein (1968), Sheridan (1973) and Hellbrügge and von Wimpffen (1975). These milestones are largely statistical, with great individual variations due to culture, nutrition and other factors. It is necessary, however, to understand *why* a baby can do certain things at certain times; why he can roll over, sit up, sit, crawl, stand up and walk only at certain stages of maturation and development.

The answer is that the maturation of the brain allows certain basic abilities to develop, and the child is then able to use them for overt functional activities. A study of these basic abilities—the result of increasing brain maturation—and their gradual development, will prove valuable not only for diagnosis and early recognition of cerebral palsy, but—more important still—will give valuable additional information for an assessment of the baby's treatment requirements, and for a re-evaluation of response to treatment.

CHAPTER 2

Normal Postural Reflex Mechanism

Fundamentally, the function of the central nervous system (CNS), with respect to our motor behaviour, is to give us the ability to move and perform highly skilled activities while maintaining our posture and equilibrium. Every movement and every postural change will produce a shift of the relationship of the body's point of gravity with respect to the supporting ground. Thus if we are not to fall, there must be an almost fluid change and fluctuation of the tonus throughout the body musculature in order to maintain our balance while moving or performing a skill. These adaptations of the tonus involving the total body musculature are constantly changing, and dynamic patterns are brought about automatically. During these adaptive changes to preserve our equilibrium whilst moving, the central nervous system is constantly activating arrays of muscles in patterns of co-ordination, in which individual muscles lose their identity: 'There is no one known muscle in the body we can throw into action separately and independently of the collateral effects of others.' (John Hunter as cited by Beevor 1903.) Jackson (1958) said that the brain knows nothing of muscles, only of movement.

Man's evolving ability to resist gravity required the solution of two contradictory problems. On the one hand, 'muscle tone' throughout the body musculature had to develop sufficient tension to give the necessary resistance to the increase of the pull of gravity, but it could not be too great and had to give way to an intended movement in a controlled manner. Phylogenetically, the first rather unsuccessful attempt by nature at solving this problem may have been to produce an abnormal static condition with poor mobility. This is borne out by the neurophysiological fact that decerebration in the cat or the dog, as produced by Bazett and Penfield (1922) and Sherrington (1947), resulted in 'decerebrate rigidity', a state of hypertonus which gave the animal the ability to stand, but at the expense of the necessary dynamic balance and righting mechanisms to maintain this state against disturbing influences, *i.e.* an exaggerated 'static' ability (Pollock and Davis 1927). In fact, this is exactly what spasticity is—a point that will be returned to later. However, man had to move in many and varied ways, and to perform highly skilled activities. For this purpose he gradually developed a highly complex automatic mechanism, the so-called 'normal postural reflex mechanism'. This mechanism, which gives us the prerequisite for normal functional activity, is responsible for the evolution of three factors:

(1) *A normal 'postural tone'*. The term 'postural tone' rather than muscle tone is used to give expression to the fact that, for the purpose of control of posture and movement, muscles are activated in patterns in which single muscles lose their identity.

(2) *The great variety of interaction of opposing muscle forces by reciprocal innervation*. This results in the simultaneous contraction of opposing muscle groups,

especially around the proximal parts, hips and shoulders, and is called co-contraction. This, through dynamic fixation of the proximal parts, allows us selective and skilled distal activity: for instance, manipulation controlled by the relative fixation of shoulders, and also the ability to stand on one leg while walking. Also, the proper integration of the action of agonists, antagonists and synergists which give power and strength to an intended movement, such as cocking the wrist for a powerful grip.

(3) *The great variety of patterns of posture and movement that are the common heritage of man.* This is demonstrated by the similarity of the fundamental sequences of the development of motor mechanisms in the maturing infant. It also finds expression in the similarity of our defence reactions under stress; for instance, the parachute reaction of which we make use when in danger of falling, and which may result in a typical injury, such as a Colles' fracture or dislocation of an elbow.

Aspects of these three factors should always be considered together as an expression of the normal postural reflex mechanism. They are not established at birth but develop in a fairly typical sequence in step with the maturing CNS.

The normal postural reflex mechanism consists of two groups of automatic reactions—righting reactions and equilibrium reactions—which in the adult are fully developed and integrated to form what has been called by Schaltenbrand (1925, 1927) 'principal motility'. This is because they are the background against which all purposeful and highly skilled activity takes place. They have been studied by Magnus (1926) and Rademaker (1931, 1935) in animals, and in man by Schaltenbrand (1926, 1927), André-Thomas (1940), Rushworth (1961) and Peiper (1961). Equilibrium reactions and their development in the growing infant have been described by Weisz (1938) and Zador (1938).

Righting reactions

The righting reactions are automatic but active responses, which not only maintain the normal position of the head in space (face vertical, mouth horizontal) but also the normal alignment of head and neck with the trunk and of the trunk with the limbs. In restoring the normal alignment of the head and neck with the trunk, they give man one of the most important features of human mobility; that is, rotation within the body axis, between the shoulders and pelvis. For all our movements are in reality rotatory and even our joint surfaces are obliquely orientated. It is the particular merit of Kabat (1952, 1958) that he stressed this aspect of human motility, pointing out that rotatory patterns of movement alone are often effective in the cerebral-palsied child to counteract hypertonus. This is because one of the factors lacking in these children is rotation between shoulder and pelvis and vice versa.

What is meant by the alignment of trunk and limbs? The baby from three months onwards has developed the 'placing reaction' of the arm and hand by placing it palm down for support. In all other activities of the emancipated limb the child looks into his palm. This is man's normal alignment of trunk and limb, although children and even adults may return to the simian type of support on the back of the hand when under stress. This type of support is most commonly met with in athetosis and in some spastic diplegias. Milani-Comparetti (1964, 1965), perhaps rightly, would call some of the 'righting reactions' de-rotatory, as the rotation serves to restore a disturbed alignment to which we always return automatically.

Head control
Another important function of the righting reactions, both for physical and mental development, is to give man head control and the maintenance of the normal position of the head in space. From about six months onwards, the child controls his head well and maintains its normal position, face vertical, mouth horizontal. As will be shown, this control of the head is one of the most important features initiating any activity against gravity from supine and prone, and is also an important feature of human communication. Initially, our orientation in space is purely subjective. 'Left' and 'right', 'above' and 'below' are really initially referring to our own head position as the fixed point from which the eyes look into space. They only become communicable later on by the fact that we all have the same head position in space to which we always automatically return.

These important physical abilities and mental concepts are assured by the interplay of five groups of reactions:
(1) the neck righting reaction;
(2) the labyrinthine righting reaction on the head;
(3) the body righting reaction on the head;
(4) the body righting reaction on the body;
(5) the optical righting reaction.

The optical righting reaction (that is, righting by vision) should be separated from the first four. Although righting by vision becomes dominant in all higher organisms, it can only be fully active after the remaining righting reactions have achieved the normal head position in space and in alignment with the rest of the body. Since this does not usually take place in a child with cerebral palsy, vision is not a great help to these children in the control of normal alignment. It may tell him that he is not aligned but he cannot correct it as long as his movements are controlled by abnormal patterns of hypertonus or co-ordination.

In normal circumstances all these groups of righting reactions interact with one another very closely and cannot be seen in isolation. The individual reactions can only been seen in experiments on animals, or by following their development in the growing infant as they come into play.

Demonstration of righting reactions in animals
In his animal experiments, Magnus (1924) placed the dog or cat in a so-called 'zero position', removing their labyrinths by a special technique of fast centrifugation, blindfolding them and holding them in the air with information by touch on both flanks. Thus the animal was devoid of any visual information, and symmetrical touch and proprioception were minimal. The head hung down under the influence of gravity and was not brought into alignment with the body. Magnus then removed the blindfold and the animal's head immediately assumed the normal position, the face vertical and mouth horizontal. The animal maintained this position in space as if held

7

by a magnet. This showed righting by vision (*the optical righting reaction*).

In a blindfolded animal placed in the zero position, but with intact labyrinths, the action of the labyrinths led to a righting reaction on the head, probably due to the interaction of the two otolithic organs (*the labyrinthine righting reaction on the head*).

If a blindfolded animal with no labyrinths was lowered from the zero position, so that any part of the body or the paws came into contact with the table-top, the head again immediately assumed the normal position in space (*the body righting reaction on the head*).

This head righting, however, produced a misalignment of the head and neck with the trunk, leading to a rotatory righting movement of the trunk into alignment with head and neck (*the neck righting reaction*).

The body righting reaction on the body was tested by moving the blindfolded and labyrinthless animal on its side into contact with the table-top, but restraining the head while allowing the trunk to move; the trunk assumed the normal posture. If the head was then released it also became aligned, again showing the effect of the neck righting reaction.

It can be seen, therefore, that in this very important righting function, tactile, labyrinthine, proprioceptive sensations and vision each play their respective rôles, one often compensating for the lack of function of another. It should also be noted that three of these reactions are rotatory, stressing the great importance of rotation and de-rotation for all motor activities.

Equilibrium reactions

The equilibrium reactions are highly integrated and complex automatic responses to changes of posture and movement, aimed to restore disturbed balance. They require for their proper functioning the contribution of the cortex. They manifest themselves in either very slight changes of tone throughout the whole body muscu-lature, detected only by palpation or electromyography, or in visible, automatic counter-movements to restore the disturbed balance. They can be tested in two ways: either by moving the body against a fixed support, or by placing a person on a balance board. In the first example, the type and extent of an equilibrium reaction depends on the speed of handling by the examiner and also on where he holds the person, and how much support he gives.

Righting and equilibrium reactions are closely integrated in the normal adult from about three or four years of age, at which time the righting mechanism becomes part of all the equilibrium reactions. In the process of integration, some righting reactions become partially inhibited, and may disappear alto-gether. Thus the adult man reaches a state where he can control and maintain the normal head position in space, and also maintain his equilibrium without the help of his arms and hands. The postural reflex mechanism in man reaches a degree of perfection which allows him to maintain his posture and balance his head, trunk and lower extremities in all ordinary circumstances, while arms and hands remain free for skilled manipulative activity. To do this, the equilibrium reactions closely interact with the righting reactions, making possible the maintenance of the head position in

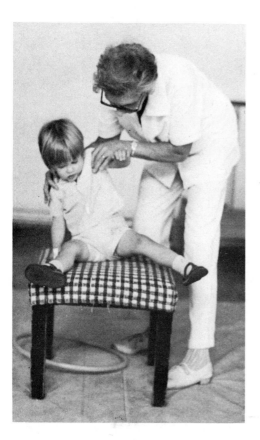

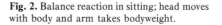

Fig. 2. Balance reaction in sitting; head moves with body and arm takes bodyweight.

space, and using the rotatory ability in their balance activities.

Man has two possible defences against the forces of gravity. If he gradually moves out of balance, his head will retain its normal position in space, and trunk and lower limbs will maintain the balance. If the balance is upset suddenly, man will make use of the parachute reaction of the arms as a second line of defence and the head may or may not move with the body. Figures 3, 4 and 5 show typical equilibrium reactions in kneeling, standing and sitting. Fig. 6 shows the parachute reaction in standing (and see Figure 2 for parachute reaction in sitting).

A simple test to find out when the righting reactions are fully integrated with the equilibrium reactions has been described by Schaltenbrand (1927). The child is asked to lie on his back on the floor and then made to stand up. As long as the righting reactions are still dominant, the child will do this with rotation. Up to about 18 months he will turn to prone before standing up. This gradually disappears to give way to the adult form of symmetrical standing up at about five years of age *i.e.* when equilibrium reactions are functional (although there is great individual and racial variation in this).

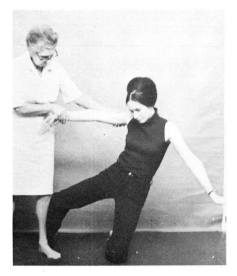

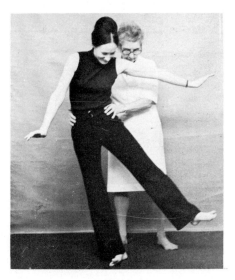

Fig. 3.   Fig. 4.

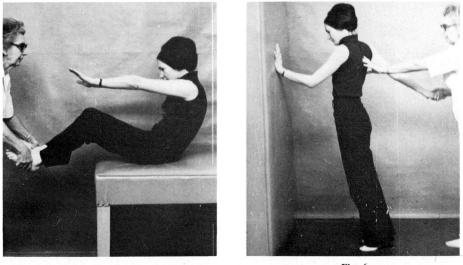

Fig. 5.   Fig. 6.

Fig. 3. Equilibrium reaction in upright kneeling; head retains normal position but trunk flexors tense on right, with abduction of limb on that side.

Fig. 4. Equilibrium reaction in standing. Normal Head position is maintained and limbs are abducted on left side when body is pushed to right.

Fig. 5. Balance in sitting; head is maintained in normal position while arms and trunk move forward.

Fig. 6. Parachute reaction if equilibrium reaction fails. Head moves in line with body and arms still 'give' despite co-contraction.

CHAPTER 3

Important Aspects of Normal Motor Co-ordination

Normal development is characterised by the gradual maturation of postural control with the appearance of righting, equilibrium and other adaptive reactions. These form the background of normal skilled activity. This process is closely integrated with the modification of the total primitive motor synergies, and culminates in the liberation of arms and hands from the necessity of playing an essential part in the maintenance of balance, except in emergency. This enables man to develop the manipulative skills to a high level of perfection. The description of this development will stress this aspect rather than give the usual account of child growth. It will not be a full account of normal development but rather describe only certain aspects which seem to be of particular value in early recognition, assessment and treatment of children.

The neonatal period

The newborn baby is not a reflexive being, as stated in some accounts of his behaviour (Peiper 1961), but shows great variability of motor patterns. Although the cortex is still immature, it already seems to exert a definite influence on the motor activities of the newborn. The normal baby shows variable behaviour, with some underlying, fairly predictable and stereotyped reflexes. It is therefore better to speak of the baby's 'automatic reactions'* rather than 'reflexes', to give expression to their variability and potentiality of adaptation to the different demands of the environment.

The newborn at rest shows a fairly symmetrical attitude of flexion or semi-flexion of trunk and limbs in all positions. He will be flexed, therefore, in supine and prone (Fig. 7a and b), ventral or dorsal suspension (Fig. 8a and b), and in vertical suspension with the head or feet up (Fig. 9). This is due to a physiological hypertonus of the flexors of trunk and limbs of fairly symmetrical distribution. The arms will resist passive extension and when released will spring back into flexion. This may be due to the absence of the 'antagonistic inhibition phenomenon' described by Gatev (1972); that is, the absence, during the first two months, of the anticipatory inhibition of an antagonist prior to activating the agonist. Head control is poor but not absent, and if the baby is placed in prone he will raise it, at least intermittently (Prechtl and Beintema 1964, Prechtl 1977) and turn it to one side (Fig. 7b) (Illingworth 1960). The baby will also turn his head freely from side to side in supine, following an object held up to about 20cm away. When following with his eyes he may show incomplete co-ordination, with an alternating squint. On observation he may also show a great deal of activity, depending on his general state of alertness (Prechtl 1965). The hands will move freely to the mouth or upper chest, with the hands and even individual

*Some authors use the word 'responses'.

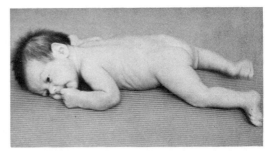

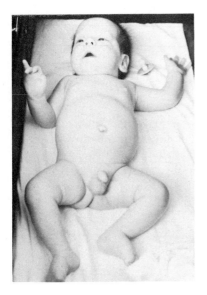

Fig. 7. Normal baby at two weeks in supine (*a, left*) and prone (*b, above*): note head turned to the side.

fingers opening and extending, but with relative inactivity of the thumbs.

The baby has no asymmetrical tonic neck reflex but, at most, an occasional attitude of asymmetrical tonic neck reflex (Gesell 1938). A study of 108 healthy newborn babies between the first and sixth days by Vassella and Karlsson (1962) has shown that in only nine of them (eight per cent) could the asymmetric tonic neck reflex be observed with the regularity of a true reflex; however, even then it does not interfere with the symmetry of the trunk and the baby's ability to get either hand to his mouth. It may become more frequent later on as the baby extends, but will disappear around the end of the fourth month.

The fingers do not only show a true grasp reflex but a 'tonic grasp of the finger flexors', as André-Thomas and Saint-Anne Dargassies (1952) and André-Thomas *et al.* (1960) rightly stress, a proprioceptive response to stretch of the flexor muscles of the hand (Fig. 9a). This seems to be relic of arboreal life, and is a reaction which is still active in the young monkey, enabling him to cling to his mother while she uses

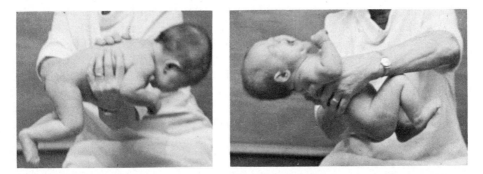

Fig. 8. Normal baby at two weeks in ventral suspension (*a, left*): note degree of head control; and in dorsal suspension (*b, right*): note poorer head control than in ventral suspension.

12

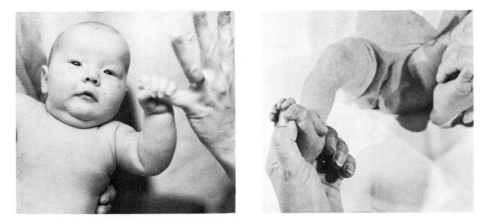

Fig. 9. Normal baby at two weeks showing tonic grasp of finger flexors (*a, left*) and grasp reflex of foot (*b, right*). (By courtesy of Dr. I. Flehmig.)

both hands for tree climbing. A rudimentary grasp response to tactile stimulation of the plantars is also present in the feet (Fig. 10*b*). Arms and hands also resist passive extension but will open widely in the Moro reflex (Fig. 11*a* and *b*). This is obtained by pushing the baby up to sitting with the examiner's hands behind the baby's head (Fig. 11*a*), then releasing the head and catching it again after a slight drop. This also results in an abduction of the legs. The Moro reflex should be differentiated from a similar reaction—the startle reaction—which occurs either for no recognisable reason, or as a result of anything startling the baby, such as a noise or cold air. Bench *et al.* (1972) define the startle reaction as a generalised 'paroxysmal' response, involving the whole body in a relatively diffuse way, whereas the true Moro is more specific. Of practical importance, however, is the fact that the true Moro can be used to test the degree to which a baby has acquired head control, as it is obtained by letting the head fall into extension. It is modified and disappears around four months when the head

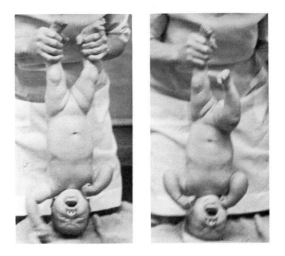

Fig. 10. Normal baby at two weeks in vertical suspension (*a, left*). Note that leg falls into flexion when released (*b, right*).

13

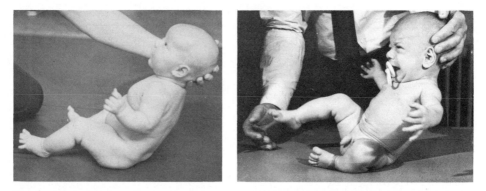

Fig. 11. Normal baby at two weeks pushed to sitting. (*a, left*) Note good abduction of arms and legs. Dorsal spine is relatively extended and hips are well-flexed. (*b, right*) Moro reflex, showing close association of upper and lower extremities.

ceases to drop back because of better control. It is, therefore, not surprising that it may be retained as a primitive feature in many children with cerebral palsy who have poor head control.

The arms are usually less mobile than the lower limbs, the fingers open both singly and together, and even the index finger extends, while the thumb remains relatively adducted and inactive. The hands move freely to the chest and mouth, regardless of any asymmetric tonic reflex influence.

The legs show an alternate kicking pattern with moderate abduction, and the ankles are flexed and inverted. Even in kicking, however, the legs do not fully extend at the hips; in fact true hip extension comes very late, probably not before the end of the second year. Hip extension, phylogenetically speaking, is a human achievement not obtained even in the highest ape. In the newborn the hip joint is steep and shallow, and this, together with the hormonal softening of the ligaments of the joint, commonly results in hip dislocation, and also makes early hip dislocation in a child with cerebral palsy possible. The hip joint develops its depth and the protection of the upper shelf through the stimulation of kicking and standing. If these stimuli are lacking, as is frequent in the child with cerebral palsy, the hip will remain dysplastic and the adduction pattern may cause subluxation or dislocation which is seen frequently in cerebral palsy. This is often the result of immobility, due to either hypotonia or spasticity. Another factor adding to the possibility of dislocation is the usual asymmetry of the condition. Early treatment with stimulation of the hip by putting the child on his feet may prevent this (Lesigang and Schwägerl 1974).

Righting reactions

Of all the righting reactions, only the neck righting reaction is present in the neonatal period. If the baby's head is turned to one side, and one waits long enough, this will be followed by a rotation of the trunk following the head in toto (Fig. 12). The baby will turn to that side. The labyrinthine righting reaction acting on the head is very immature and weak. It will allow the baby to raise the head for a short while in prone, but not yet in supine. Optical righting is absent.

14

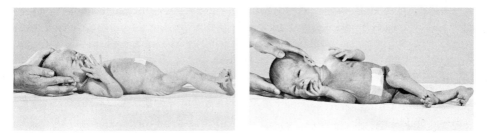

Fig. 12. Normal baby at two weeks showing neck-righting reaction. (By courtesy of Dr. I. Flehmig).

Equilibrium reactions

Equilibrium reactions are absent, nor is there any need for them, as the baby has hardly any activity against gravity. If the baby is placed in supine or prone on a table which is then tilted to one side, he will roll over towards the lower end without any preventive reaction (Weisz 1938).

Other automatic reactions

In the full-term newborn during the first few weeks these include: (1) the Galant reaction; (2) the placing reaction of the feet; (3) automatic primary standing and walking; (4) the reaction of the baby to being pulled by his arms into the sitting position (also called traction response); and (5) the rooting reaction, already mentioned.

(1) GALANT REACTION (THE TRUNK INCURVATION REFLEX) (GALANT 1917)

This is tested with the baby lying in the prone position or in ventral suspension. A blunt pin is drawn down the skin of the lumbar region between the 12 rib and the iliac crest paravertebrally. This leads to a lateral flexion of the trunk towards the stimulated side (Fig. 13). According to André-Thomas *et al.* (1960) this reaction will normally disappear during the second month. However, Ingram (1962) observed

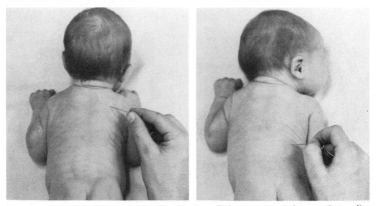

Fig. 13. Normal baby at two weeks showing Galant or trunk-incurvation reflex; stimulation (*left*) and response (*right*). (By courtesy of Professor H. F. R. Prechtl).

15

it in babies three months of age. This reflex seems to denote an instability of the trunk of the baby, closely associated with lack of head control and the general flexion of the trunk. In a child with cerebral palsy, and especially in the unstable athetoid with poor head control and inability to extend the spine in prone, it is frequently persistent for much longer. Its retention may cause considerable delay in the development of symmetrical stability of the trunk and of independent movements of the head necessary for sitting, standing and walking. This may also sometimes happen in diplegic children and may make sitting difficult due to an unstable trunk, in spite of fair head control. The disappearance of the Galant reaction seems, therefore, to coincide with the gradual extension of the spine in prone, initiated by the improved head control. In my experience it disappears around the end of the third month when the process of trunk extension and stability reaches the lower ribs.

(2) THE PLACING REACTION OF THE LEGS

This is obtained by suspending the baby vertically and gently bringing the anterior aspect of the legs or dorsum of the foot into contact with the edge of the table (Fig. 14a). The baby will flex the leg and bring the foot above the surface of the table. This will be followed by extension of the legs so that the sole of the foot touches the surface (Fig. 14b). According to André-Thomas et al. (1960) this reaction is obtainable after the first 10 days. Prechtl and Beintema (1964) found that the reaction was not pronounced during the first four days.

The statement that the absence of the placing reaction denotes a severe degree of mental subnormality (Foley et al. 1964, Zappella 1964) must be accepted with great reservation, as it may be absent in children with severe degrees of extensor spasticity of the legs, regardless of the degree of mental retardation.

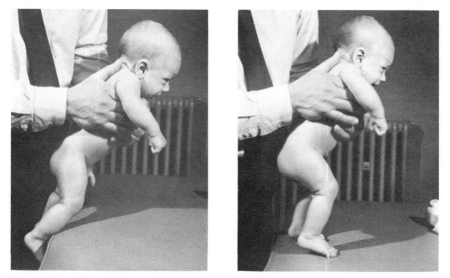

Fig. 14. Normal baby at two weeks showing placing reaction of the legs. Stimulation (a, left) and response (b, right).

(3) PRIMARY STANDING AND AUTOMATIC WALKING

Primary standing is obtained by placing the baby with his feet on the table. He will gradually right himself and assume the standing position. This righting ability disappears during the second month (André-Thomas and Saint-Anne Dargassies 1952, André-Thomas *et al*. 1960). According to Peiper (1961) the assumption of the 'primary' standing posture in the neonate is the result of the positive supporting reaction of the legs.

Automatic walking can be elicited by placing the baby with his feet on a table while the examiner supports the baby's unstable trunk with both hands under the axillae. The baby will first right himself and assume the standing position. If during this righting the body is now tilted forward, the baby will begin to walk with well co-ordinated and rhythmical steps (Fig. 15). He raises the legs high, and does not extend either hip or knee fully. The equilibrium and stability of the trunk necessary for maintaining the erect posture are absent. If support of the trunk is withdrawn the baby will slump over to one side. This walking may persist for a variable period of up to two months. However, according to MacKeith (1964), it can still be obtained in most babies under one year of age by combining the above-described manoeuvre with passive extension of the baby's head.

An interesting phenomenon has also been described by André-Thomas and Autgaerden (1966). This is the ability of the baby during automatic walking to continue over an obstacle placed in his way. This led the two authors to discuss the question as to whether the baby is aware of the obstacle, a problem that remains unanswered.

(4) THE TRACTION RESPONSE (PULLED TO SITTING) (FIG. 16a-c)

If the baby is pulled from supine to sitting his head will drop back. The degree to

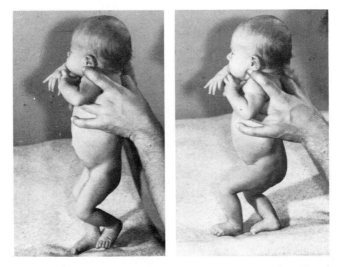

Fig. 15. Normal baby at two weeks showing development of automatic walking. Note that the trunk has to be well supported because it is still very unstable at this time. (By courtesy of Professor H. F. R. Prechtl).

17

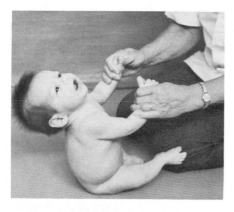
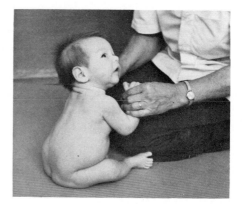

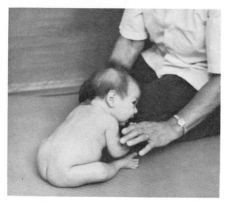

Fig. 16. (*a, above left*) Normal baby at two weeks pulled to sitting; (*b, above right*) at about 80° from horizontal the head comes forward; and (*c, left*) from the sitting position, baby slumps forwards into flexion.

which it does so within normal limits is a matter of experience. If the pull is stopped when the baby is almost vertical, he will slowly bring his head up into alignment with the trunk. On shaking the baby the head will, however, ballot fairly freely. From sitting, the baby slumps forward into flexion (Fig. 16c).

If the baby is pushed up to sitting with the examiner's hand at the back of the head, the baby will come up with a relatively straight dorsal spine and well flexed hips

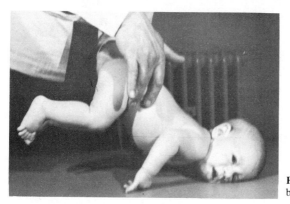

Fig. 17. Normal baby at two weeks lifted by pelvis; legs are flexed and mobile.

18

(see Figure 11*a*). If from there the head is allowed to drop back a little before being caught again, the arms and legs will abduct widely in the aforementioned Moro reflex. This shows an important fact of normal development: that abductions of arms and legs are closely associated.

If the pelvis is lifted off the support in prone, the legs will remain flexed and mobile (Fig. 17).

General remarks

The baby will turn his head freely in supine and prone, following a sound, or a visual stimulus if it is not held too far from his eyes. He can move his hands to his mouth and upper chest but cannot as yet reach out and grasp an object. If he is held feet down and with his back against the examiner's chest, and if the examiner *then* turns away from a source of light, the baby's eye movement will lag behind—the Doll's eye syndrome. Conjugate movement of the eyes will be poor and the baby shows a physiological transient squint. Sitting control is poor, head righting and equilibrium reactions are absent (Fig. 18).

From 1 to 10 months

There is no other period of postnatal development as fast as that during the first year. The maturation of the labyrinthine righting reaction of the head, probably closely associated with the maturing cerebellar-cortical systems, results in the fast improvement of head control during this period. As a general rule in the development of the righting mechanism, prone development is ahead of supine control of gravity.

Prone development

The baby begins to raise his head more consistently in prone from about four or five weeks onwards. This leads to a gradual extension of neck and spine, a process which advances cephalo-caudally. At about two months* the baby is able to raise his head well in prone and rest on his forearms (Fig. 19). The increase in extensor tone

*All time sequences should be taken as approximate as there are wide individual variations.

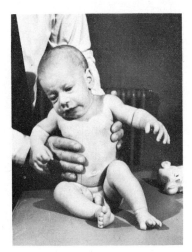

Fig. 18. Normal baby at two weeks showing absence of balance and head-righting if pushed sideways.

19

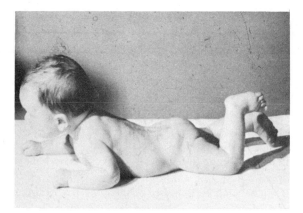

Fig. 19. Normal baby at two months showing improved head control. Note support on abducted forearms.

involves the spine cephalo-caudally and at about three months, when it reaches the rib region, the Galant reaction disappears (the gradual extension of the trunk is closely associated with an increasing stability and symmetry of the trunk). At about this time the placing reaction of the arms and hands develops. If the baby is moved in horizontal suspension so that his forearms come into contact with the edge of a table, he will raise the arm and place his hand on its surface, palm down (Fig. 20).

As the extension in prone initiated by the raising of the head reaches the lumbar region and leads to further extension of the hips, at about four months the kicking pattern changes. The baby now kicks not only in a total flexion-abduction pattern but also with an isolated knee flexion-extension pattern; that is, independently of the hips, both unilaterally and bilaterally. This kicking pattern is with extension, outward rotation and from medial to lateral. Head control is also more stable and he can play with an object near his body in prone at five months. At five to six months the legs are externally rotated, extended and abducted. However, he can only maintain his head position in total extension (Fig. 21) and if he attempts to get on all fours, for instance, can do so only by flexing his head, and his position will change to

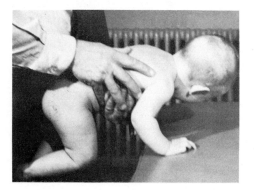

Fig. 20. Normal baby at three months showing placing reactions of the arms and hands (normal alignment, palm down).

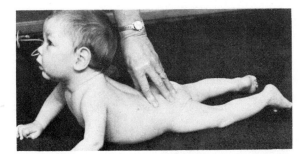

Fig. 21. Normal baby at five months in prone, showing full extension with arms in abduction and legs abducted and rotated outwards.

one of general body flexion (Fig. 22). At this stage he therefore shows a *primitive total extensor pattern* against gravity when in the prone position. He can now take his weight on his extended arms, resulting in the development of the parachute reaction. In the prone position he is able to follow an object from side to side with raised head while supporting himself on extended arms, but he cannot reach out for the object as he still needs both arms for support. This extension finds expression in the Landau reaction (Fig. 23). If the baby is held in ventral suspension supported under the lower chest and upper abdomen by one hand, he will raise his head followed by a symmetrical tonic extension of trunk and hips. If the baby's head is passively flexed the body and hips will also flex and if the head is tipped sharply downwards towards a surface the baby will extend his arms forward in the parachute reaction (Fig. 24). In some babies a Landau will be present as early as four months.

Now that the baby has developed fair head control, extension, and with it a measure of activity against gravity, the early equilibrium reactions develop, first in the prone position and soon after in supine, at about seven months. For instance, if a baby of about six months of age is placed in prone on a table which is then raised at one end, the baby will show a definite and logical defence reaction. The muscles on

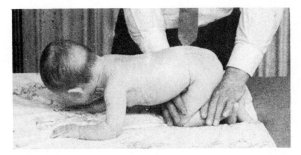

Fig. 22. Normal baby at five months showing total flexion with loss of head control when legs are flexed; as yet, unable to get onto all fours.

21

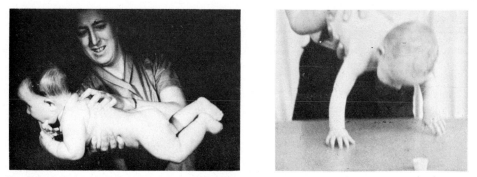

Fig. 23 (*left*). Normal baby at five months showing Landau reaction. Note the relative extension of the hips only.

Fig. 24 (*right*). Normal baby at 10 months showing parachute reaction forward. This reaction is active from about five months throughout life.

the upper side of the baby's trunk will contract, arching the body upwards. The head will move into alignment with the trunk and the upper limbs will abduct.

Supine development towards sitting and the assumption of the standing posture

Gradually, the baby will also extend in supine. As he extends, the asymmetric tonic neck reflex, though still occasional, will become more frequent (Fig. 25). Essentially, development is characterised by the gradual increase of head control. This enables the baby to initiate activity against gravity to an increasing degree. From

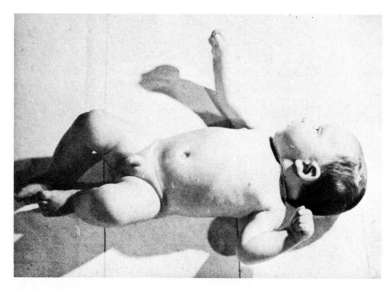

Fig. 25. Normal baby at two months showing asymmetric tonic neck response. It is most commonly seen at this age but only as an occasional attitude. It does not interfere with the ability to bring other hand round to mouth or body and does not produce asymmetry of trunk.

22

about three months onwards, when the baby is pulled to sitting the head will initially fall back but will come forward when the baby is about 30 or 40 degrees from the horizontal. As he is pulled to sitting, his legs will lift off the support, first in flexion-abduction and soon after in extension-abduction. The improved head control finds expression in the gradual modification and final disappearance of the Moro reflex, which at about two months becomes a reaction of abduction of the arms, associated with flexion of the elbows, and disappears around the fourth or fifth month with the appearance of forward propping, which I regard as the parachute reaction (Fig. 26). The baby therefore develops, around the fourth or fifth month, with the help of the developing righting mechanism, a total, normal but primitive extension pattern against gravity in prone, and a total, normal and primitive flexion pattern against gravity forward from supine.

An important point is that in this development of anti-gravity control from supine forward, the upper dorsal spine is relatively more extended than the flexed lumbar spine and hips. This picture is often reversed in the spastic baby, a point which will be taken up later.

At about five months the baby will now reach out and forward with an open hand, and the tonic grasp of the finger flexors is replaced by a true tactile grasp response. He will also be able to play with his body lower down, reaching the lower abdomen.

Equilibrium reactions

The first equilibrium reactions in supine and prone develop at about six and seven months, when the baby can already maintain the sitting position if put there. They overlap with the righting reactions. This overlap of developmental abilities is an important factor to take into account in the treatment of children with cerebral palsy. It shows that a treatment programme that follows the developmental sequence too strictly in terms of perfecting one activity, such as sitting and kneeling, before proceeding to standing is physiologically unsound and may result in the development of undesirable effects, such as flexion contractures of hips and knees. Even in terms of purely functional development it is well known that some babies may skip some

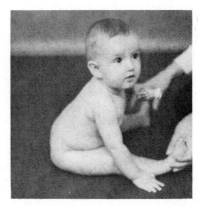

Fig. 26. Normal baby at about six months, sitting. Note parachute reaction forward.

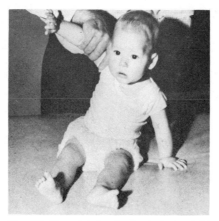

Fig. 27. Normal baby at about six to eight months showing sideways arm support when sitting.

activities, such as crawling, completely.

At about five months, head and trunk control are well established. If the baby is now pulled to sitting, even by one hand only, the head will come forward immediately and the baby will assist in sitting up. He will sit fairly freely but still rely on the parachute reaction to either side (or lateral propping) to maintain the sitting posture (Fig. 27).

From about seven months onwards, the baby adopts a fully extended posture in prone, with good abduction of arms and legs. The primitive total rotation pattern of the neck righting reaction is now modified by the appearance of the body righting reaction acting on the body. The baby now acquires the skill to rotate within the body axis, between shoulders and pelvis, and will soon turn from supine to prone and vice versa. He will also be able to sit up, which the normal baby does for at least the next two years by first turning from supine to prone. The ability to extend and rotate in prone, together with the now-established equilibrium in prone, allows the baby to shift his body weight onto one extended arm and rotate the body to set one arm free to reach into space (Fig. 28). The baby begins to play with his feet and explore them with his mouth in supine (Fig. 29).

At about eight months the Landau reaches its climax, kicking stops, the grasp

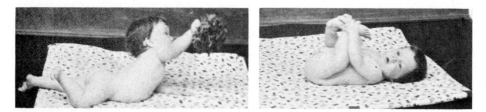

Fig. 28 (*left*). Normal baby at about eight months. Full extension and abduction of limbs makes rotation possible. This, with equilibrium in prone, frees the arm to reach into space.
Fig. 29 (*right*). In supine the baby of seven to eight months plays with his feet and brings them to his mouth.

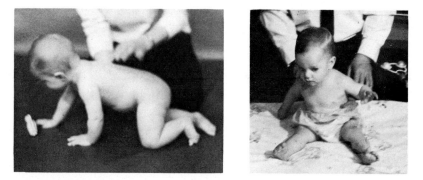

Fig. 30 (*left*). Normal baby at about eight months can now move on all fours without flexing his head.

Fig. 31 (*right*). By 10 months there is good equilibrium in sitting on a wide base; arms are almost free from the necessity of supporting and can be used for manipulation.

response of the feet stops (Illingworth 1960) and the baby is now well prepared to learn to stand. In sitting, the first equilibrium reactions begin at a time when the baby is already pulling himself up to standing. Closely integrated with the perfection of head control, rotation and equilibrium, there begins a process of modification of both the earlier total extension and flexion patterns. The baby can soon go on all fours and crawl while maintaining his head position without flexing it (Fig. 30). In sitting he can combine flexion of the hips with extension of the spine in such a way as to use the arms for lateral support (around six to eight months) (Fig. 27) and later for support behind him (10 to 12 months). Soon the perfection of the equilibrium reactions set arms and hands free for manipulative activity (Fig. 31). From about six or seven months the righting reactions become progressively integrated with the equilibrium reactions and the process of integration will go on for the next five years.

Schaltenbrand (1926, 1927) has described a simple test to show when the righting mechanism is wholly integrated with the equilibrium reactions. As long as righting reactions are still active, the child will only be able to stand up from supine by rotating into prone; the infant up to two years or older will therefore not be able to stand up from supine without first turning into prone. This rotation gradually disappears and from about four or five years onwards the child will stand up in the adult symmetrical fashion.

CHAPTER 4

The Application of Normal Child Development to the Assessment of the Child with Cerebral Palsy

Co-ordination of movement for skilled activity needs many years of orderly development. One has to appreciate that motor development is not a separate entity but profoundly influences all other aspects of the child's behaviour. As already mentioned, learning is based on sensorimotor development. It begins with the child's exploration of his own body. He learns about his mouth, lips and tongue through touch by his hands, and his hands also play with each other. He will learn about textures, shapes, temperatures and objects by touching and sucking them. He learns about his own size when reaching out for objects, when crawling over and under furniture. The ability to move and to adjust himself increasingly to changes of posture means safety and comfort. Righting and equilibrium reactions develop, enabling him to get himself out of uncomfortable positions. The child's perceptual and visuomotor development is profoundly influenced by his physical development. Abercrombie (1960, 1968) and Rosenbloom (1971, 1975) have found that limitations in the child's capacity for active movement retard the unfolding of his perceptual abilities, and in this way interfere with his over-all intellectual capacities. The interaction of movement with speech development has been stressed by many workers, for instance Luria (1961). Children speak with movements and gestures long before expressing themselves verbally, a habit to which even the adult returns when in a foreign country, without an adequate knowledge of that language. Speech and manipulation are important features of the thinking process and delay in speech development may seriously affect abstract thinking ability.

The child with cerebral palsy cannot make himself independent from his mother's support. He remains dependent upon her not only physically but also emotionally and intellectually. This exaggerated dependence is established often in earliest childhood and may become so marked as to interfere with the potential abilities of the handicapped child. Metaphorically speaking, it seems that in some of these children the umbilical cord was never severed.

We learn through sensations; we do not learn a movement but the sensation of a movement. A child, whether normal or abnormal, can only use what he has experienced before. The normal child will use and modify his normal motor patterns by practice, repetition and adaptation. The child with cerebral palsy will continue to use and, by repetition, to reinforce abnormal motor patterns. He will build new abnormal compensatory patterns based on his earlier abnormal ones. He will thus have to function without the help of many of the sensorimotor patterns which a normal child acquires very early on in life and which should have provided him with the foundation for the more complex and difficult tasks of mature life (Held 1965, Denner and Cashdan 1967, Hellebrandt 1977).

The child with cerebral palsy, therefore, has two major disadvantages: (1) insufficient normal faculties with which to develop functional skills; and (2) abnormal sensorimotor experience on which to base future development.

It is important to appreciate that it is insufficient in the treatment and management of these children to manipulate the sensory input, important as it is for the child's intellectual development. This by itself will only result in an inadequate and abnormal output of the damaged brain. It is, in fact, the bright, active and well-motivated child who seems most in danger of developing contractures and deformities if he is made to use his abnormal patterns with effort.

The assessment of the nature of the handicap of the child with cerebral palsy purely in terms of an interference with the attainment of the usual milestones is not sufficient. As already stated, developmental scales are purely descriptive. They give a 'longitudinal' picture of development, only stating that a child can do certain things at a specific time. Furthermore, they are largely statistical, with wide individual variations, as Illingworth (1960) rightly stresses. More valuable in this context are studies of the French school (André-Thomas and Saint-Anne Dargassies 1952, André-Thomas et al. 1960) and of the Groningen school (Prechtl and Beintema 1964, Prechtl 1977), as they have studied the neurological factors of this maturational process. The most valuable tables, however, in the context of the assessment of the child with cerebral palsy, are the scales of McGraw (1963) and especially the studies by Touwen and Prechtl (1970) and Touwen (1976), as they take into account the great overlap in the appearance and disappearance of certain automatic reactions and reflexes, giving optimal times for their activity and their gradual fading in and out. Although still statistical, they are a better guide to assessment, lending themselves to a cross-sectional study of the developing motor abilities. This point will be returned to later. Touwen also stresses the fallacy of a strict adherence to the so-called three monthly period of neurological maturation, and of interpreting minor deviations as pathological and in need of treatment. For the assessment of the child and subsequent development of a plan of treatment, we should think, therefore, more in terms of the development of motor co-ordination. One has not only to describe the acquisition of an ability at a certain time but, as stressed earlier, to explain the reason why a baby can only do a certain thing at a certain time. What are the underlying factors in the maturing brain which get translated into observed functional activity? A knowledge of development in these terms has proved of immense value for early recognition and classification of children with cerebral palsy, and has also given valuable clues for treatment, evaluation and reassessment of results.

CHAPTER 5

Tone and Posture in the Assessment of Cerebral Palsy

A lesion of the brain will interfere with the working of the normal postural reflex mechanisms and can interfere with three factors of normal postural control (described in Chapter 2) in various ways: (1) instead of a normal postural tone the child may show hypertonus; that is, spastic or plastic hypertonus; or he may show the intermittent spasms of the majority of the athetoid group of cerebral palsy; (2) instead of the normal degrees and variety of reciprocal innervation, the child may show abnormal deviations, the type of disturbance depending on the site of the lesion; and (3) instead of the great variety of the normal patterns of posture and movement, the child will show abnormal patterns of co-ordination due to the release of abnormal postural reflexes (the so-called static or tonic reflex mechanisms of Magnus) with either fixation, as in a few typical patterns of spasticity, or abnormally exaggerated mobility with lack of fixation, as in the athetoid group.

Abnormal postural tone

This is classically examined by passively moving the different segments of a limb and testing the resistance of the muscles to passive stretch. It is unfortunate that, so far, modern neurophysiology has not been able to explain the different types of abnormality of muscle tone seen in the different types of cerebral palsy. However, a certain amount is known about the nature of spasticity. It is considered to be a release of the gamma system, and more rarely the alpha system, from higher inhibitory control (Rushworth 1960, Boyd *et al.* 1964). Presumably the release of a facilitatory mechanism within the reticular substance of the brainstem enhances the sensitivity, or 'bias', of the gamma system. This then becomes hyperexcitable and reacts to a 'normal' stretch in a 'maximal' manner, resulting in a synchronised total discharge of all anterior horn cells to a muscle group. The result is a synchronised excitatory phase (Magoun and Rhines 1946, 1948), followed by a synchronised post-excitatory phase of inhibition (Sherrington 1913). After the passing of this phase a new wave of post-inhibitory excitation returns. This may explain the clinically observed characteristics of spastic muscle—an exaggerated stretch response, the clasp knife phenomenon, and the lengthening and shortening reactions. More difficult to explain is the 'rigidity'. This term, originally introduced by Sherrington (1947), is unfortunate. It is very different from the rigidity observed in Parkinson's disease. It is, in fact, a very severe degree of spasticity, produced by maximal release of the gamma system from higher inhibitory control. Rigidity in cerebral palsy, better named 'plastic hypertonus', is recognised by the unchanging resistance of a muscle group to passive stretch throughout the whole range of either flexion or extension (The Little Club 1959). This may be the result of exaggerated co-contraction; that is, the opposition of fairly evenly matched spastic muscle groups, which happens in severe spasticity, usually around the proximal joints, the shoulder girdle and hips.

There is no satisfactory explanation yet for the nature of the intermittent spasms seen in many of the athetoid types of cerebral palsy. The amplitude of fluctuation of tone may vary widely in the individual case, either with a base of poor postural tone or at the most a normal tone. Flaccidity of postural tone is usually a transient phenomenon in cerebral palsy, occurring in early infancy and followed sooner or later in most cases by a spastic or plastic hypertonus, or the unstable and fluctuating tone characteristic of the athetoid group. The explanation for this type of postural tone may be a high threshold of the gamma system to stimulation, due to an overactive inhibitory system of the brainstem (Magoun and Rhines 1946) released from cerebellar control. These children may show considerable increments of tone under sufficiently strong, long-lasting or repetitive stimulation.

A more permanent type of hypotonia is characteristic of cerebellar ataxia. This is due to a more permanent lack of inhibitory control by the cerebellum. Ingram (1954, 1964) has described typical cases of diplegia with generalised ataxia associated with spasticity of the lower extremities. This is presumably due to a lesion which interferes both with the control of the higher facilitatory and inhibitory centres of the brainstem and with the interaction between the cerebellum and the corticopontocerebellar connections.

Myotatic responses

The assessment of the type and strength of the myotatic response to stretch may be of some value in the diagnosis and classification of cases of cerebral palsy. It is, however, of little value in working out a programme of treatment and assessing its results, for the following reasons.

First, hypertonus and hypotonus as muscular phenomena are very variable, changing with the child's general condition and excitability and with the strength and speed of stretch. Secondly, different types of abnormalities of tone may be observed in the same child in different parts of the body. Thirdly, the type of abnormal tone in an affected part may change in time as the brain matures. This will necessitate reassessment and reclassification of a case (this applies especially to the infant who is initially 'floppy'). Fourthly, as will be shown later, the strength and distribution of hypertonus in any particular part of the body will change with alteration of head position in space, or with the position of head and neck in relation to the trunk (due to tonic reflex activity).

Spasticity can be viewed as a local muscular phenomenon with a neurophysiological explanation. This view had influence on the treatment of this condition until about 35 years ago and led to a predominately orthopaedic approach to treatment. Spasticity was looked upon as static and unalterable, and treatment encouraged the child to make the best use of his handicap by compensation with less affected parts. Physiotherapy attempted to increase the range of motion at certain points by passive stretch, subliminal in strength in order to avoid strong stretch responses. Orthopaedic measures were aimed at tiring out stretch reflexes by bracing, and also sought to prevent undesirable deformities by transfer of tendons, neurectomies, and by surgical correction of deformities once they had occurred.

Reciprocal innervation and inhibition

An understanding of the law of reciprocal innervation—the second factor of postural control—and of the type of disturbance caused by an abnormal interaction of opposing and muscular forces, may be of great value in differentiating the various types of cerebral palsy and offer valuable clues to treatment. It will also go some way to explaining the reasons for the imbalance of opposing muscular forces which the orthopaedic surgeon finds so difficult to assess, and also to predict the result of an intended operation. These problems have been discussed by Pollock (1955), Blundell Jones (1961), Sharrard (1961), Tardieu (1961) and Samilson (1975).

Sherrington (1913) stressed the importance of reciprocal innervation for the regulation of postural tone in the maintenance of equilibrium and the performance of normal movements. He showed that in a spinal animal, in the flexor withdrawal reflex the agonists were excited and contracted while simultaneously the antagonists were relaxed by central inhibition. He called this phenomenon 'reciprocal inhibition'. He stated that inhibition was an active process exerted by the central nervous system. He further stated that 'reciprocal inhibition' as observed in spinal animals was an artefact—a very special case of 'reciprocal *innervation*' and not likely to occur in normal circumstances.

In normal circumstances the modifying influence of higher centres on the spinal mechanism of reciprocal inhibition from brainstem, midbrain, cerebellum and cerebral cortex resulted in the agonists, antagonists and synergists being pitted against each other in a far more adaptable manner of reciprocal 'innervation' than occurs in simple reciprocal inhibition. The antagonists are inhibited and relaxed in a finely graded adapted manner, in step with the contracting agonists. They therefore exert an important steadying and guiding influence on the movement in progress. Synergistic muscle groups contract to steady and fix neighbouring joints, giving precision to the moving part and optimal mechanical conditions for power and strength resulting from the regulation of the interplay of opposing muscular forces. For instance, in a contraction of the finger flexors, as in grasping an object, the extensors relax while the synergists raise the wrist and stabilise it in an extended position. Sherrington also showed that in certain circumstances both the agonists and the antagonists were in a state of simultaneous excitation and contraction by reciprocal innervation. This is especially relevant in postural control, as when standing on one leg, or when fixing the shoulder to support precise movements of the hand and finger. In normal circumstances this simultaneous contraction of opposing muscular forces by reciprocal innervation, called 'co-contraction' by Riddoch and Buzzard (1921), is however, of a moderate and controlled degree, allowing for mobile fixation.

In the child with a spastic or plastic type of hypertonus there seems to be on the one hand a deviation of reciprocal innervation towards an excess of co-contraction (see Table I), in which spastic muscles oppose equally or more spastic muscles (this is especially marked at proximal joints of the hips and shoulder girdle), and on the other hand there may also be a deviation towards an excess of reciprocal 'tonic' inhibition, wrongly called 'weakness' of a muscle, through inhibition by spastic antagonists (for instance, the so-called 'weakness' of the tibialis anticus with loss of isolated dorisflexion of the ankle when the leg is in a total spastic extension-adduction pattern). It can be shown that this is not true weakness, as the ankle dorsiflexes easily if the leg is flexed in a total flexion-abduction pattern, and cannot, in fact, be actively extended.

These two types of deviation can be seen simultaneously in the same spastic child in different parts of the body. For instance, it may be found that all the muscles around the shoulder girdle are in a variable degree of spastic co-contraction with a depression of the shoulder and fixation of the shoulder blade, and that there is resistance of the arm to active or passive elevation, to extension backwards, to movements forwards, and to horizontal abduction. Further examples are the simultaneous spastic contraction of the flexors and extensors of the hips with resistance to their full passive or active extension or flexion, and the equinovarus of the ankles due to 'weak' peronei in opposition to spastic tibiales anticus and posticus.

Co-contraction in the moderately spastic child may not be evident until the child attempts to move, when the effort will make him stiffen his limbs owing to the increased spasticity and associated reactions and simultaneous contractions of agonists and antagonists. For instance, an attempt to raise the arm will only result in a further accentuation of depression of the shoulder. Spastic or plastic hypertonus and the disturbance of reciprocal innervation seem to explain the immobility (relative or absolute) of spastic children, their fixation in a few typical abnormal patterns, and their difficulties in moving. Spasticity therefore results in an exaggerated static position, with loss of the normal stato-kinetic reactions of the normal child. The child suffers fundamentally not from weakness of muscles but from an impoverishment of movement patterns. Movements, if at all possible, will be limited in range and direction and require excessive effort.

In the ataxic and athetoid group of children the deviation of reciprocal innervation seems to be towards an excess of reciprocal 'inhibition' (see Table I), the degree of deviation varying in the individual child. Any attempt at a movement will lead to excessive relaxation of the antagonists. The lengthening group of muscles are unable to guide and hold the movement. Lack of co-contraction is also responsible for the poor supporting action of the synergists. This explains the excessive mobility and lack of fixation and postural control of this group of children. Their movements are characterised by poor control, extreme ranges, and poor co-ordination. This seems

TABLE I

Reciprocal innervation and deviations in different types of cerebral palsy

EXTREME ◄——————— NORMAL ———————► EXTREME	
Reciprocal inhibition	*Co-contraction*
The spastic child (distal reciprocal tonic inhibition) The ataxic child The athetoid group The floppy infant	The spastic child (exaggerated co-contraction proximally)

31

to be the reason why Hammond (1871*b*) gave the name 'athetosis' to this condition, meaning 'no fixed posture'. The two factors described so far, that is the abnormal postural tone and impaired reciprocal innervation, important though they are, can only be considered in conjunction with the prevailing abnormal patterns and their influence on normal activity.

Abnormal patterns of muscular co-ordination

The third and most important factor in the assessment of handicap in the child with cerebral palsy is the abnormal patterns of muscular co-ordination, both in posture and movement, and their interference with normal postural control, balance and functional skills. While strongly agreeing with Milani-Comparetti (1964) that a study of the patterns of co-ordination is of utmost importance, giving as it does valuable clues to assessment, re-assessment and planning of treatment, the two factors mentioned above (abnormal muscle tone and reciprocal innervation) cannot be disregarded altogether because they give important additional information.

It is perhaps not surprising that Milani-Comparetti places almost exclusive emphasis on the study of patterns of posture and movement, as his concepts are based on the study of young babies with cerebral palsy. In these infants abnormal qualities of postural tone are not yet clear and the main problem of treatment, therefore, is one of 'reconstruction' of patterns following the developmental sequence, rather than the necessity to inhibit abnormal patterns of hypertonus and facilitate normal motor patterns. This is also borne out by Milani-Comparetti's developmental assessment chart, which is of great value in making a quick assessment, and as a preliminary screening of babies who show developmental retardation rather than obvious abnormality.

CHAPTER 6

Tonic Reflexes

The tonic reflexes of particular relevance in cerebral palsy are:
(a) the tonic labyrinthine reflex;
(b) the tonic neck reflexes: (i) asymmetrical and (ii) symmetrical;
(c) associated reactions (Walshe 1923);
(d) the positive and negative supporting reactions.
These reflexes have been explained in great detail in previous publications *e.g.*
Hochleitner 1968, 1969; Flehmig 1979; and Bobath (see Reference List).

A knowledge of the individual tonic reflexes is of help in analysing the motor deficit of children with cerebral palsy. However, their influence should not be overrated since they are only rarely seen in isolation, as are the abnormal patterns in their pure form. Furthermore, they are reflexes which have been studied predominantly in decerebrate animals. The interpretation of the motor behaviour of the child with cerebral palsy therefore should not rely solely on trying to trace these few abnormal reflexes and their interaction. The motor patterns of the cerebral-palsied child are the result of the interplay of all these various abnormal reflexes, and also of the factors of which we are less aware, resulting from the injured human brain.

It is comparatively easy to see these reflexes at work in a severely spastic or athetoid child, who most clearly shows released 'tonic reflex' activity, since the spasticity and intermittent spasms are often too strong to allow any modification of the primary abnormal patterns by compensatory activity. In most cases, however, the reflexes and the patterns of movement are changed in time by the child's compensatory activities, which are themselves abnormal but cannot be interpreted only in terms of the primary reflexes. The child's effort produces secondary abnormal patterns of greater individual variety; it is therefore far more important to study the patterns of hypertonus, both primary and secondary compensatory, as they show themselves in the individual child, regardless of whether they can be explained in terms of the few known 'tonic reflexes' and their interaction. Furthermore, it is most important to assess the manner in which they interfere with normal balance and functional ability.

We have observed, over a long period, considerable changes in the condition of children with cerebral palsy in this and other developed countries. The tonic reflexes, for instance, as described in previous publications, are rarely seen in their pure form. However, they can still be observed clearly and their interplay studied in the severely palsied and older children whom we now see from the developing countries. The disappearance of the pure tonic reflexes in the developed countries may be due to the improved care, treatment and management of these children and especially better training of their parents. Furthermore, we see many more atypical cases of cerebral palsy among the 'floppy infant' group in particular.

I feel that in the past I may have overrated the significance of the 'tonic reflexes', probably to the detriment of credibility in this approach to treatment. However, that does not materially change the fact that hypertonus is an abnormal, patterned response of the damaged central nervous system, and that the logical treatment of spasticity is by inhibition of these patterns. Further support for the pattern theory is given by animal experiments. In a cat or dog, the lesion which produces the release of spasticity also produces the pattern of 'standing against gravity', the animal being able to stand but unable to maintain the standing position against disturbing influences because of the loss of the righting mechanism. Decerebration of these animals frees the centres of facilitation and inhibition within the brainstem: these regulate normal postural tone by modifying the interplay of alpha and gamma activity in the spinal cord (Wilson 1920, Magoun and Rhines 1946). The release of these brainstem centres within the reticular substances leads to overactivity of the various tonic and static reflexes. They are called 'tonic' reflexes since they are the cause of hypertonus, and 'static' because they make the animal excessively static, with a loss of the adaptable stato-kinetic reactions of the midbrain and thalamic animal.

Tonic labyrinthine reflex

This abnormal reflex is evoked by changes in the position of the head in space, which stimulate the otolithic organs of the two labyrinths. This reflex is never seen in man in normal circumstances, but only in association with spasticity or intermittent spasms. It is not a primitive reaction and is not seen in normal babies as has been frequently stated in the American (Snell 1976)) or German (Flehmig 1970, 1979) literature. As the labyrinths are fixed within the head, it is the position of the head

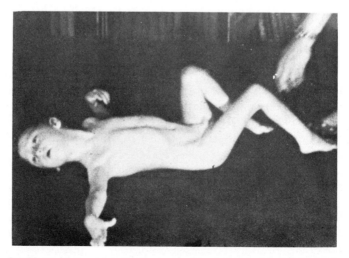

Fig. 32. Spastic quadriplegia showing combined picture of tonic labyrinthine reflex and asymmetrical tonic neck reflex. Note secondary semi-flexion contractures of lower extremities, severe co-contraction preventing full extension and flexion of these extremities.

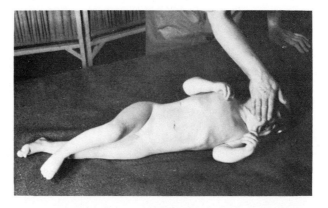

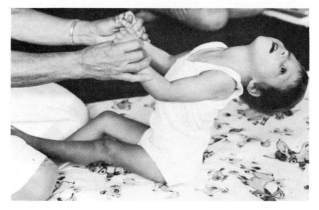

Fig. 33. Spastic quadriplegia; difficulty in turning to one side because of retraction of right shoulder.

Fig. 34. Child with spastic quadriplegia pulled to sitting (traction response). Note poor head control.

itself which determines the distribution of hypertonus throughout the affected parts. In the totally involved quadriplegic patient the reflex usually causes maximal extensor hypertonus in the supine position with the head in the midline, and minimal extensor hypertonus with a relative increase of flexor hyperactivity in the prone position. This means that most quadriplegic patients, both spastic and athetoid, experience great difficulties in initiating any activity against gravity in supine or prone.

In spastic quadriplegia (Fig. 32) there is retraction in supine of the head, neck and shoulder, the trunk is stiffly extended and the legs are adducted and inwardly rotated, with plantiflexed ankles. The chest is usually expanded as a result of the extensor position, the mouth is open and the child has difficulties in exhaling. This is the typical picture of primary severe spasticity, which will remain unchanged only if the condition is so severe that the child cannot of his own accord change the abnormal positions and adapt them to give a degree of functional ability. The child is unable to lift his head, he cannot bring his trunk forward and flex his hips; therefore he is unable to initiate sitting up. He cannot bring his arms forward to grasp an object or to help pull himself into the sitting position, nor can he bring his hands to his mouth or to any other part of his body. The rigid contraction of the trunk and the shoulder retraction make rolling over, even to one side, difficult or impossible (Fig. 33) and if

35

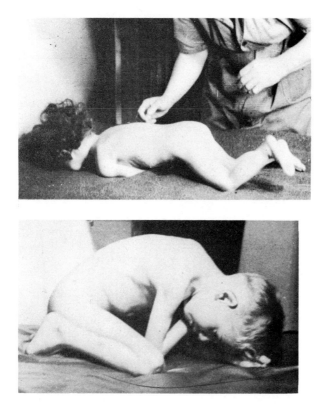

Fig. 35. Spastic quadriplegic lying in prone. Note total flexion of head in midline so that child has difficulty in breathing.

Fig. 36. Spastic quadriplegic child kneeling. Note lack of head control and arm support.

he is pulled by his arms into the sitting position his head falls back (Fig. 34).

When lying in prone and kneeling, the child shows strong flexor hypertonus (Figs. 35 and 36). Head, shoulder and spine are flexed, sometimes with the head fixed in the midline. The arms are adducted, one or the other being caught under the body. The spine is rounded, and the hips, knees and ankles are flexed and sometimes abducted. However, it sometimes happens that the hips are extended; then the legs will also show a pattern of total extension and adduction, with plantiflexion of the ankles. The child is unable to lift his head, to extend the spine or to free the arm caught under his body; he cannot push himself up into extension and cannot look forward. If he is lifted up the arms will pull up in flexion (Fig. 37). He cannot get himself into a kneeling position on all fours, nor can he turn to sit.

If the hypertonus is very strong it will not only interfere with the child's motor activities but will also hinder cognitive development, which depends on the child's ability to move and to explore himself and his environment. The poor head-control prevents the child from looking around, and from normal babbling, sucking, chewing and speech development. This point has been rightly stressed by Rosenbloom (1971), who underlines the close inter-relationship of physical, intellectual and emotional pathways in the infant's developmental processes. The same point is also made by

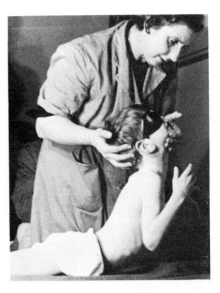

Fig. 37. No arm support by child with spastic quadriplegia when lifted up from prone.

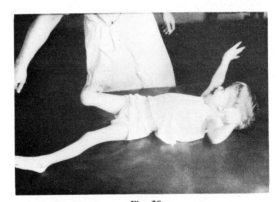

Fig. 38. Athetoid quadriplegic showing (a) intermittent tonic labyrinthine reflex producing extensor hypertonus in supine; (b) dystonic attack, opisthotonic attitude. (c) Athetoid child in supine.

Fig. 38a

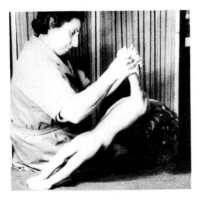

Fig. 38b

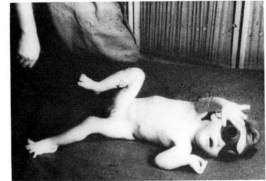

Fig. 38c

37

Abercrombie (1960, 1968).

In most children with cerebral palsy the extensor tone is most pronounced in the supine position and flexor hypertonus is most pronounced in the prone position, probably due to the influence of the tonic labyrinthine reflex. However, there are exceptions, depending on the child's initial type of hypertonus. Some quadriplegic children with severe extensor spasticity and opisthotonus in supine may still have strong extensor hypertonus in the prone position, although to a lesser degree. Some children may show strong initial flexor hypertonus which may still be prevalent in the supine position, although again to a lesser degree.

The subsequent development of abnormal patterns in different types of cerebral palsy will be described in greater detail later.

The athetoid child with intermittent spasms will tend to show extensor spasms when attempting to move in supine (Fig. 38 *a, b, c*) and flexor spasms when attempting to move in prone (Fig. 39).

The early inability of the normal baby to raise his head in supine does not indicate an active tonic labyrinthine reflex, but rather the still-existing immaturity of the normal postural righting mechanism. This is borne out by the fact that the normal newborn baby is already able to raise his head in prone. A child with an active pathological tonic labyrinthine reflex cannot raise his head either in prone or supine. Furthermore, the tonic labyrinthine reflex is always associated with typical patterns of abnormal hypertonus.

Asymmetrical tonic neck reflex

This is a proprioceptive response obtained from the muscles of the neck and probably also from the ligaments and joints of the cervical spine. Turning the child's head to one side will increase extensor hypertonus on the side to which the head is turned (the face side) and flexor hypertonus of the opposite side (the occiput side). This does not occur as an obligatory reflex in the normal baby: turning the head may result in an occasional extension of the arms but will not interfere with the symmetry of the trunk and lower limbs. Furthermore, it will not affect the free movement of arms and hands to the mouth or chest.

The pathological asymmetrical tonic neck reflex is associated with the extensor pattern of cerebral palsy. It will occur in both athetoid and spastic patients: when sitting, if the child tries to look up and extensor spasticity or spasm supervenes, the child is in danger of falling backward. It also occurs in standing when the spastic or athetoid child is extended. The normal asymmetrical tonic neck reflex also occurs more regularly with extension and therefore is not conspicuous even as an attitude in the flexed or semiflexed early state of the newborn. It will become more frequent from about four or six weeks after birth as the baby begins to extend in the supine position, and will finally disappear around the fourth month of life. The normal asymmetrical neck response will not interfere with the symmetry of the trunk, nor will it prevent the baby from turning his head from side to side or from sucking his fingers.

This reflex in the cerebral-palsied child may affect the whole body and be responsible for producing considerable asymmetry. In a severe case of quadriplegia (both spastic and athetoid) with intermittent spasms, the result of head-turning may

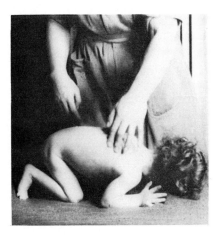

Fig. 39. Athetoid child kneeling, showing flexor spasms in prone.

Fig. 40. Athetoid quadriplegic showing asymmetrical tonic neck reflex (*a*) in supine; (*b*) in sitting; and (*c*) in standing.

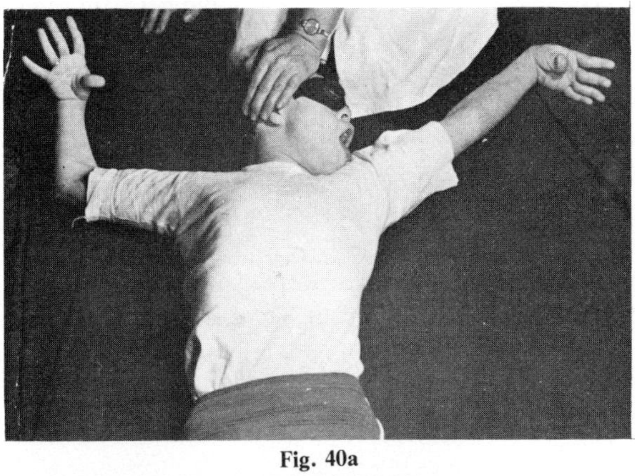

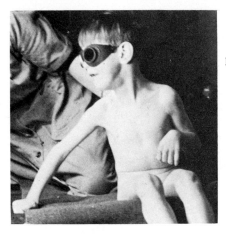

Fig. 40a

Fig. 40b

Fig. 40c

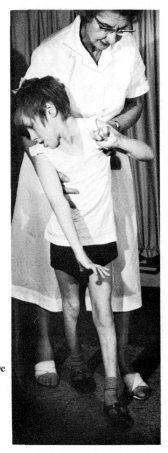

be almost immediate, especially when associated with extension imposed by the tonic labyrinthine reflex, *i.e.* in supine, sitting and standing, when the head is extended and tilted to one side (Fig. 40 *a, b, c*). In milder cases there may be a latency period of varying length, depending on the effort, speed or difficulty of moving the head. In some diplegic children the effect may only be seen in the lower extremities: as one side of the child is usually more involved than the other, the effect may be stronger on the more affected side, or only be seen on that side. The head is then often turned to one side, and can only with difficulty be turned to the other side. It must be appreciated that an asymmetrical distribution of hypertonus may also occur, without an obvious asymmetrical tonic neck reflex.

The asymmetrical tonic neck reflex may prevent the child from reaching out for and grasping an object while looking at it. In order to grasp the object the child has to turn his head away from it: the arm will then be brought up to the back of the head (the occiput). He cannot bring hand and fingers to his mouth; not infrequently, his eyes are fixed toward the face side and he cannot move them across the midline.

The asymmetrical tonic neck reflex is usually stronger and more immediate toward the right, so most children with this reflex will appear to be left-handed. The dangers of the asymmetry, whether as a result of an asymmetrical tonic neck reflex or of different involvement of the two sides, will be discussed later.

Symmetrical tonic neck reflex

This is also a proprioceptive response evoked from the proprioceptors of the neck muscles by an active or passive movement of raising or flexing the head. Raising the head produces an increase of extensor hypertonus in the arms and flexor hypertonus in the legs. Lowering the head has the opposite effect.

When the child with cerebral palsy is placed on his knees he usually shows a total picture of flexion and cannot extend his arms. However, if his head is passively raised he may extend his arms but his legs will be fixed in flexion, owing to the influence of

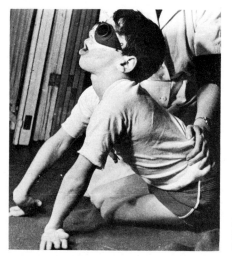

Fig. 41. Athetoid quadriplegic showing symmetrical tonic neck response.

the symmetrical tonic neck reflex (Figs. 41 and 42). Some children in whom the symmetrical tonic neck reflex is stronger than the tonic labyrinthine reflex cannot kneel with their head down, because their legs then extend and their arms flex (Fig. 43). If the legs are passively flexed they may assume a total flexion-abduction pattern (Fig. 44).

The severely affected quadriplegic child usually shows so much flexor hypertonus when lying prone that he cannot get up to the kneeling position. In this case the tonic labyrinthine reflex dominates. The less-affected quadriplegic and the diplegic children may get themselves into the kneeling posture by making use of the symmetrical tonic neck reflex pattern. They can therefore sit on their heels with the head raised and take their weight on extended arms, but they cannot extend their lower limbs at hips and knees to get into a kneeling position on all fours, or move

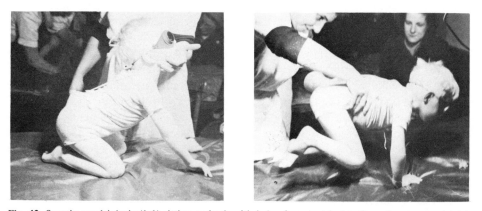

Fig. 42. Spastic quadriplegic (*left*) sitting on heels with help of symmetrical tonic neck response; (*right*) with head raised, arms are almost able to carry bodyweight and legs are locked in flexion.

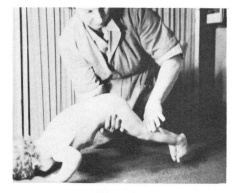

Fig. 43. Spastic quadriplegic showing symmetrical tonic neck response with the head down; arms are flexed and legs extended and adducted, resisting flexion.

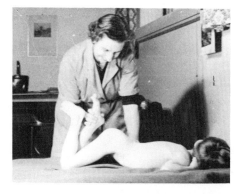

Fig. 44. Spastic quadriplegic in prone. If legs are passively flexed, overcoming spastic resistance, they flex in a total flexion-adduction pattern (competition of patterns).

them alternately as in crawling. They may look fairly normal when sitting on their heels, but can only progress on the flexed lower limbs by pulling themselves forward with the help of their arms. When pushed to sitting their arms and trunk will flex and the legs will extend and may even cross (Fig. 45).

The combined effect of the labyrinthine reflex and of the asymmetrical and symmetrical tonic neck reflexes on a child with spasticity, or on the intermittent spasms of the athetoid quadriplegic child, will be discussed later.

Associated reactions

Associated reactions are perhaps the most important of all the abnormal tonic reflexes, being responsible more than any of the others for the development of contractures and deformities. They are tonic reflexes spreading from one limb to the rest of the affected parts (Walshe 1921, 1923). In the child with cerebral palsy they produce a widespread increase of spasticity in all parts of the body not directly concerned with the intended movement. In the quadriplegic child the effort of moving one limb will increase hypertonus in the rest of the body. Associated reactions must not to confused with 'associated movements', which we all tend to have when doing anything with great effort, and which also occur in normal circumstances when learning a new skill. This happens especially in children; for instance, when trying to write for the first time. The child will contort his face with the effort and often show mirror movements in the other hand. However, associated movements are never stereotyped and never occur in the same unchanging patterns as do associated reactions: they have the variety of normal patterns. Associated reactions, on the other hand, are stereotyped, always working into the same unchanging patterns of spasticity. They produce increased spasticity which may result in a visible accentuation of the abnormal posture, or be discovered only by palpation. In this constantly increasing spasticity, with increasing co-contraction and accentuation of the abnormal posture, lies the danger of their eventually producing permanent contractures and deformities. The occurrence of associated reactions is well illustrated in a child with a spastic hemiplegia (Fig. 46). At rest in the standing position she shows a left-

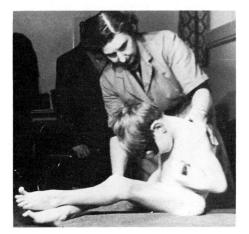

Fig. 45. Spastic quadriplegic child with some athetoid features showing symmetrical tonic neck response when pushed to sitting. Such children may be able to sit on a stool with extended legs and flexed trunk and may be able to use both hands near the body but not be able to reach out.

sided hemiplegia with initially moderate spasticity. She is made to squeeze a rubber ball with the sound hand; the result is a strong increase of spasticity with accentuation of the abnormal posture. The same effect of increased spasticity is also obtained by asking the child to lift the hemiplegic leg, and an even more severe effect results from asking the child to try to stand on the affected leg. Associated reactions are induced by fear, lack of balance, and effort, and there seems to be a direct relationship between strength of effort and severity of resulting increase in spasticity. The same effects can be obtained in spastic diplegia and quadriplegia: in the former, the spasticity of the usually mildly affected arms and hands can be considerably increased by lack of balance in sitting, standing and walking, caused by fear and undue effort. Therefore, during treatment one should not make the child use any part of his body with effort, because in trying to improve the function of a single affected part one may make the rest of the body worse. Treatment must always take into account the whole of the condition.

Positive supporting reaction

The positive supporting reaction is the static modification of the spinal extensor thrust, making a limb into a rigid pillar of co-contraction for weight-bearing (reflex standing). It is produced by a twofold stimulus:
(1) Tactile; that is, by the touch of the ball of the foot on the ground.
(2) Proprioceptive; that is, by pressure resulting in a stretch of the intrinsic muscles of the foot.

As a result, postural tone in the lower limbs increases in both the flexor and extensor groups of muscles (co-contraction; Pollock and Davis 1927) but more so in the anti-gravity muscles. The leg stiffens and becomes a rigid pillar for support. The

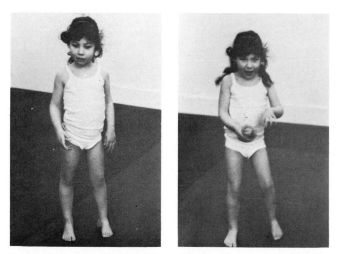

Fig. 46. Child with left hemiplegia at rest (*left*), with little weight on left leg and moderate spasticity; (*right*) squeezing ball with normal right hand, there is a shift of bodyweight away from left leg, and increased spasticity.

effect persists as long as the two types of stimuli are active.

Under normal conditions the positive supporting reaction occurs in many only in a very modified form. Standing on one leg will produce co-contraction of the muscles of that limb. However, the limb still remains mobile in all joints, and the normal child is able to flex hip, knee and ankle separately to any required degree without collapsing.

In attempting to stand, the spastic child touches the ground with his foot and exerts pressure on the foot within the reflexogenic area of the positive supporting reaction. He is prevented from putting his heel to the ground by an upsurge of extensor spasticity which produces the well-known pattern of extension, inward rotation and adduction of the whole of the standing leg, with plantar flexion of the foot. The standing base is therefore narrow and small. Pressure of the foot against the ground tends to throw the child backwards and makes weight transference onto the standing leg difficult. If he raises one leg to take a step, extensor spasticity in the standing leg will increase still further. When he puts the raised leg down again to take the body weight, extensor spasticity in the standing leg will diminish and it may flex. Both these results are due to the added influence of the crossed extension reflex on the positive supporting reaction.

The athetoid patient usually lacks a sustained extensor tone and the co-contraction necessary for standing. The positive supporting reaction is absent, and the patient uses the pattern of crossed extension reflex for walking. He can only stand on stiffly extended legs and in walking raises his legs too high in a pattern of total flexion.

CHAPTER 7

Types of Cerebral Palsy

This chapter will deal with the various types of cerebral palsy, classified according to the three factors previously described (postural tone, type of disturbed reciprocal innervation and the distribution of the condition). The influence of the abnormal postural patterns on the child's functional abilities are discussed, with a description of the changing of the primary patterns over time and the resulting contractures and deformities. An understanding of all these factors will lead not only to a better understanding of the nature of the handicap of these children but will also form the basis for a rational approach to treatment and management. The first and main objective of treatment is to give the child a more normal background of postural tone as a preparation for normal movement and balance. It may first be necessary to define the terms used here in classifying children with cerebral palsy. These are terms now generally accepted by the International Society for Cerebral Palsy (Little Club 1959) to describe the condition according to its distribution.

Quadriplegia is defined as involvement of the whole body, the upper parts being more involved than, or at least as equally involved as, the lower parts. Distribution is usually asymmetrical. If the asymmetry is very marked, these children are sometimes referred to as 'double hemiplegics'. Due to the greater involvement of the upper parts, head control is poor, as is eye co-ordination. The children usually have feeding difficulties, and some involvement of speech and articulation. Many spastics belong to this group; practically all of the athetoid children, the mixed types of spasticity with athetosis or ataxia, and the cases of cerebellar ataxia.

Diplegia is also involvement of the whole body; the lower half however, is more affected than the upper half. Head control, and control of the arms and hands are usually little affected, and speech may be normal. However, a squint, either alternating or fixed, is not uncommon. Sometimes the upper parts seem so slightly involved that the child is diagnosed as a cerebral paraplegic. Careful examination, however, will show some involvement of one or both arms and hands (a pure cerebral paraplegic is usually of a congenital hereditary type). This group consists almost exclusively of spastic children but occasionally ataxia may be associated with a spastic diplegia. The aetiology of many cases of spastic diplegia is found to be prematurity.

Hemiplegia is involvement of one side only. Practically all of them are spastic, and children with a hemi-athetosis are very rare. Cases of pure paraplegia and monoplegia are extremely rare in cerebral palsy.

The spastic child

The spastic child shows hypertonus of a permanent character, even at rest. The degree of spasticity varies with the child's general condition, that is, his excitability and the strength of stimulation to which he is subjected at any moment. If the spasticity is severe the child is more or less fixed in a few typical patterns due to the severe degree of co-contraction of the involved parts, especially around the proximal joints—shoulders and hips. Some muscles, however, may appear 'weak' as a result of tonic reciprocal inhibition by their spastic antagonists: for instance, the gluteal and abdominal muscles by spastic hip flexors, the quadriceps by spastic hamstrings, and the dorsiflexors of the ankles by spastic triceps surae. However, true weakness may develop in some muscle groups because of disuse in cases of long standing, and after prolonged immobilisation in plaster casts or apparatus. Spasticity is of typical distribution and changes initially in a predictable manner, owing to tonic reflex activity. Movements are restricted in range and require excessive effort. The primary patterns and their predictable changes through tonic reflex activity have already been described in previous chapters, as has their early development.

Although spastic quadriplegia and spastic diplegia have many features in common, and sometimes it is not easy to decide whether a child has diplegia or quadriplegia, there are nevertheless features of the two varieties of cerebral palsy which make it useful to consider them separately. The fully established case is described below, features of which are often apparent by the time a child is one year old. The problems of early diagnosis are discussed in Chapter 8.

Spastic quadriplegia

As already stated, early recognition is not usually difficult (but see the discussion on the floppy infant in Chapter 8). Both the retardation of normal development and manifestation of abnormal signs can be seen early. Sometimes, however, erroneous diagnosis of hemiplegia may be made as the more involved side may show pathology first.

Once spasticity is fully developed, the child is unable to right his head, maintain his equilibrium in any position or to use his arms and hands. Lying in supine he usually shows strong neck and shoulder retraction (see Figure 33, page 35). Neck righting is absent and rotation of the head to one side may only lead to the assumption of an asymmetrical tonic neck reflex attitude and asymmetry of trunk and limbs. Any attempt of the trunk to follow the head and so to roll over to that side is prevented by the retraction of the shoulder. The child is therefore unable to roll from supine into lying on his side. He lacks rotation within the body axis—the result of absence of the body righting reaction acting on the body—and cannot, therefore, roll over into lying in prone. Lying in prone he is usually unable to raise his head, or to use his arms and hands for support, and therefore cannot get up. The shoulders and spine are flexed and the arms also flex if the body is lifted off the support by the shoulders. Hips and knees may be flexed. However, if the thighs are extended at the hips, the legs will be extended, inwardly rotated and adducted. The feet will then be plantar flexed at the ankles. Some children are able to lift the head in prone and maintain the puppy position, the arms flexed and over-adducted, as long as the trunk and lower extremities are extended (Fig 47a). However, if they try to get onto their knees, the head flexes, as well as the trunk, hips and legs. The legs may then adduct in a total flexion pattern (Fig. 47b).

Inability to raise the head from supine prevents him from initiating sitting up.

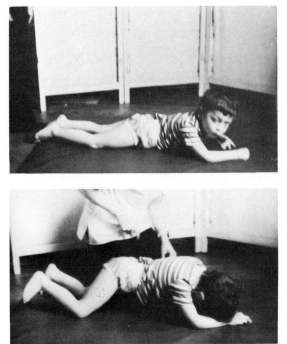

Fig. 47. Spastic quadriplegic child in prone: (*a, above*) head can only be maintained in a raised position when child is in total extension; (*b, below*) head, trunk, hips and legs flex if the child tries to get onto his knees.

He cannot bring his arms forward and into midline to pull himself up to sitting. The difficulty in sitting up is further enhanced by the inability or difficulty in flexing his thighs at his hips, which results from an increase of extensor spasticity caused by the touch and pressure of the buttocks against the support.

A few of these children develop some righting ability of the head. However, this ability is interfered with by tonic reflex activity whenever the head is moved into a position which favours its occurence. For instance, in trying to look up while sitting, the child raises his head high and will then fall backwards into extension, not infrequently throwing his arms up and out in a primitive Moro response. If head control is fair, the intelligent child may learn to avoid movements which result in tonic reflex activity. He may even learn to use his head to achieve a compromise of flexor and extensor spasticity. For instance, if flexor and extensor spasticity are strong in the supine and prone positions respectively, he may learn to sit on a stool by moving his head into a mid-position, which establishes a certain equilibrium between the two extremes of spasticity, thus allowing him to sit. He will then lean slightly backwards, compensating for insufficient flexion of his hips by dorsal kyphosis in order to bring trunk and head over the sitting base (Figs. 48 and 49). The neck will be hyperextended and the head held stiffly in a more or less normal position. The sitting base is narrow and balance precarious, owing to the adduction-flexion attitude of the legs. He cannot use his arms for support, because flexor spasticity prevents this. When attempting to raise his head, he is in danger of falling backwards due to extensor spasticity; when looking down he will slump forward due to flexor spasticity. Fig. 50

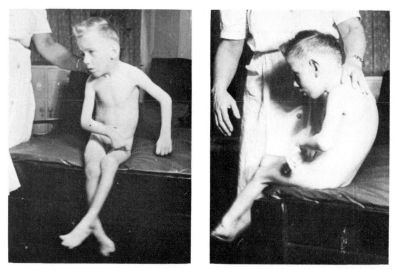

Fig. 48. Typical sitting posture of quadriplegic child needing arms for support. Note compensatory kyphosis and scoliosis.

shows the typical sitting pattern of a spastic quadriplegic. The influence of reaching out forward upsets the child's precarious balance by increasing extensor spasticity, with a danger of falling backwards. This leads to a compensatory flexion down and forwards of the head (Fig. 50).

If, in addition, the child has a strong asymmetrical tonic neck response, usually stronger to the right, he may learn to use one arm for reach and grasp by turning his head first to one side to reach out and then to the other to grasp the object. Usually the head is then turned to one side, producing asymmetry of the trunk, adding

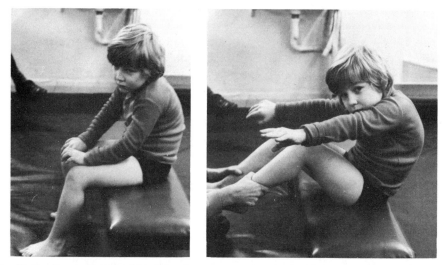

Fig. 49. Spastic quadriplegic child sitting (note compensatory kyphosis); prevents falling backward by bringing arms and head forward.

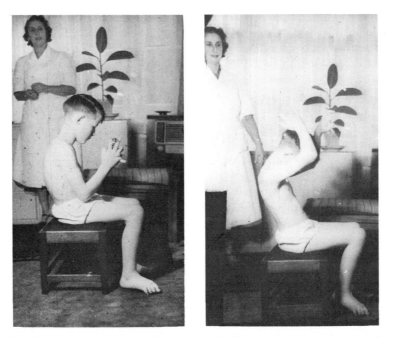

Fig. 50. Spastic quadriplegic child: a danger of falling backwards due to increased extensor spasticity on reaching forward leads to compensatory flexion of head forward and down.

scoliosis to the compensatory dorsal kyphosis (Fig 48). The child will then sit with his weight most on the more flexed hip, the pelvis is tilted, the hip joints usually dysplastic, with a danger of subsequent subluxation or dislocation of one or both hips. Sitting up and sitting on the floor with extended knees are quite impossible, due to insufficient flexion of the hips and inability to use spastic arms for support.

Other children may adopt a sitting posture of full flexion. Head and trunk are flexed forward and the child will avoid looking up in order not to fall backwards. Raising the head and turning it to one side may also produce an influx of asymmetrical tonic neck reflex in this type of spastic quadriplegia. By keeping the head and trunk well forward, the head can be controlled in the midline. However, the arms are then flexed and the child may only be able to use both arms and hands near the body, unable to extend them and to reach out, while the legs may be extended and adducted (see Fig. 45), probably due to a symmetrical tonic neck reflex. These children will eventually develop a dorsal kyphosis, with flexion deformities of the hips and knees because of a strong and persistent co-contraction of the flexors and extensors of the hips and knees.

The quadriplegic child with moderate spasticity may in time acquire some of the righting and equilibrium reactions in sitting and kneeling but not in standing or walking. Unless the child can compensate for this lack of equilibrium by using his arms and hands for support, standing and walking will be impossible. As long as the child moves slowly and carefully while sitting and avoids extreme positions, tonic reflex activity will not interfere greatly and postural tone may remain fairly normal.

The deformities likely to result from the child's use of tonic reflex patterns for functional activities may therefore be the following:

(1) A scoliosis and/or kypho-scoliosis.

(2) Flexor deformities of hips and knees, an equinovarus or equinovalgus of the ankles.

(3) Subluxation of one hip (rarely of both), usually the left hip. This may be the result of the following factors:

    (a) underdevelopment of the hip joints in a child who has never stood or walked;

    (b) adductor spasticity with a coxa vara and inward rotation of the legs;

    (c) the pelvic tilt due to the asymmetrical distribution of the condition. On the side with most flexion, spasticity of the side flexors of the trunk will pull the pelvis up and rotate it forward. This tendency is accentuated by a strong asymmetrical tonic neck reflex. This is probably the most important factor.

The factors responsible for a subluxation or dislocation of the hips in cerebral palsy seem very complex. It seems that the imbalance of muscle power between the adductors and glutei, especially the gracilis and gluteus medius, is not the whole of the problem and that the one-sided position of the child's head and the resulting asymmetry of trunk and pelvis play a major part. The main factor is, however, a dysplasia of the hip-joint, a failure of development of the so-called 'buttress' due to poverty of movement of the legs in early infancy, plus inability to stand, thus preventing the 'modelling' of the hip-joint. In early treatment this may be avoided by preparing the child for early standing, with extension of the lower extremities in outward rotation and abduction of the legs in prone on the floor or on a ball.

Spastic diplegia

During the first four or six months, the baby may seem quite normal. Signs of spasticity may be absent or only very slight. The physiological predominance of flexor tone and the baby's postural behaviour may be very similar to those of a normal baby of his age. He will develop normal head righting and, if the upper limbs are unaffected, normal parachute reactions of the upper limbs. Any abnormality will show itself only when the normal process of development of extension reaches the lower trunk and hips. If the arms are slightly involved, the protective reactions of the upper limbs will appear late and may remain incompletely developed. Head raising in the prone and supine positions may then be difficult or delayed owing to flexor or extensor hypertonus respectively.

Though the arms may not show an asymmetrical tonic neck reflex, head turning may produce tonus changes in the legs. The child may kick only with the 'occipital' lower limb, while the leg on the side to which the face is turned may be held in extension—at first in a pattern of outward rotation, but later the total spastic pattern of extension, adduction and inward rotation may develop. In the more severe cases this pattern of extension, adduction and inward rotation may develop very early, *i.e.* before the age of six months.

If the head and upper limbs are only slightly involved, or even unaffected, during the early phase of predominant flexion the child may still be able to turn onto his side. Rolling over to prone will present difficulties, however. The child will learn this much later and will be able to do it only with the help of his arms, while the lower limbs remain stiffly extended. The difficulty is largely due to a lack of rotation within the body axis and the inability to flex and bring the uppermost leg across. Once he has succeeded in rolling over to prone, he may learn to progress on his abdomen by a kind of swimming movement, *i.e.* by alternating abduction-flexion and adduction-extension movements of the lower limbs. At this stage the early, normal primitive movements of the lower limbs may still persist in the prone position, while in the supine and sitting positions the lower limbs may be in strong extension.

Later on, creeping will become impossible as extension increases and as extensor spasticity of the lower limbs simultaneously grows stronger. This happens at about the same time as the normal baby learns to extend his spine and hips sufficiently to support himself in prone on his forearms. The diplegic child will now progress by dragging himself along the floor with flexed arms and stiffly extended legs. The effort of pulling the body along in this way will increase extensor spasticity of the legs (associated reactions) and they will soon show the total extensor spastic pattern, with extensions, adduction and inward rotation.

Though the child may be able to raise his head in the supine position and to bring forward his arms for grasping, sitting up will be difficult or impossible, as his hips will resist flexion and his legs will adduct and may even cross. Sitting up may therefore be delayed up to the age of three years or longer. However, he may be able to sit with support nearer the normal stage. In such a case early diagnosis may not be made until the baby is about eight or nine months old; that is, when he should be sitting up by himself but does not do so properly and also has poor sitting balance. Fairly stable sitting is only made possible by compensating for the insufficient flexion at hip and knee joints, *i.e.* by bringing the head and spine well forward. If the arms can be extended they will be used for support, since the child lacks equilibrium of the pelvis and lower limbs (Fig. 51). The child will, at best, be able to use only one arm and hand for grasp, reach and play, and he will be unwilling to raise his head or reach

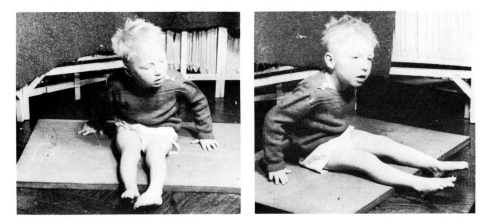

Fig. 51. Typical sitting posture of diplegic child needing arms for support.

out with both upper limbs as he will tend to fall backwards.

In some cases a persistent Moro response may add to the difficulties by making it impossible for the child to put his hands down for support to stop himself from falling backwards. The children who are unable to use their upper limbs for support behind them when sitting will compensate with flexion forwards, and the strong flexion of the spine will, in time, result in a structural kyphosis with flexor hypertonus of the shoulders and dorsal spine, and the pelvis will be tilted backwards. The original extensor spasticity at hips and knees, with relative reciprocal inhibition of the flexors, will gradually be changed into a picture of co-contraction of the flexors and extensors around the hip and knee joints. This is the beginning of the development of the well-known scissor posture of the lower limbs, later seen in standing. It will become more distinct during standing through the effect of the positive supporting reaction, which will add sufficient extensor tone for the child to stand.

The sitting pattern of the diplegic child whose upper limbs are relatively free will be different, as he can use them for support. He will use a pattern of strong flexion of the hips which helps him to abduct his thighs and flex his knees. The pelvis is tilted backwards and he sits with a stiffly extended spine. Later on, when standing up, extension at the hips becomes difficult and the child then extends his head and shoulders to assume and maintain the erect posture in spite of the hip flexion. This results in a compensatory lumbar lordosis (Fig. 52). He tends to fall backwards unless he can hold onto a support. As in the other type of diplegia, co-contraction of the muscles around the hips and knees will develop in standing and walking, with the resultant scissoring of the legs (Fig. 52).

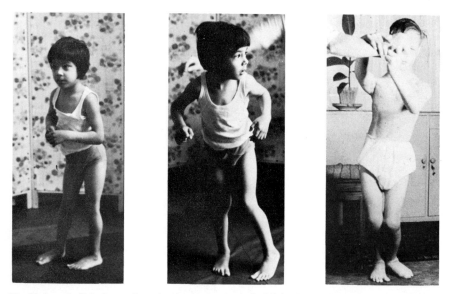

Fig. 52. Spastic diplegic standing, showing lumbar lordosis: left heel can only be placed on ground by flexing hip (shifting spasticity). Note (*far right*) typical diplegic scissor posture.

Whereas the normal child achieves a fair degree of emancipation of arms and hands around the eighteenth month, having by then acquired sufficient balance of trunk and legs, the diplegic child has to rely on his arms for support indefinitely. In early life he pulls himself along the floor, either in prone or kneeling; later, when learning to stand and walk he has to hold on to people or furniture, use sticks or crutches. This involves constant and excessive use of the flexor muscles of arms and hands and also of the shoulder girdle and trunk, which are usually involved to some extent; he will therefore retain a clumsy grasp with pronation of the forearm. This is the primitive pattern of grasp and release belonging to the earliest stages of normal child development when flexor patterns are still dominant. Extension of the hands at wrists and fingers, abduction and opposition of the thumb and supination movements of the forearm and hand will develop late and incompletely.

In standing and walking, which are acquired late and are only possible if arms and hands can be used for holding on and support, diplegic children will make excessive use of whatever righting and equilibrium reactions are present 'above the waist'. They therefore use excessive compensatory movements of head, upper trunk and arms, as the legs and hips are too stiff to take a step. They cannot shift their body weight automatically onto the standing leg in order to leave the other leg free to make a step. The body weight remains on the inside of the foot. They lack balance and rotation and seem to 'fall' from one leg to the other in walking; they are unable to stand still without holding on to something.

There seem to be two principal walking patterns:

(1) Children with strong flexion of the dorsal spine and a forward tilt of the pelvis lean backwards with their trunk in order to raise one leg and bring it forward to take a step. They then throw their body forward to transfer their weight (pigeon walk).

(2) Children who show a straight and erect dorsal spine with lordosis of the lumbar spine (due to flexor spasticity around the hips, especially of the iliopsoas) will use alternating side flexion of the trunk from the waist in order to bring the stiff legs forward. Whereas a normal person walks with mobile legs and a relatively stable trunk, these children show excessive mobility of the trunk and stiff legs.

Most diplegic children stand and walk on tiptoe, as dorsiflexion of the feet at the ankles would produce an increase of flexor tone throughout their lower limbs, making standing and walking impossible and possibly causing them to collapse. Thus, as has been mentioned before, the lower limbs of an older diplegic child will show a pattern of mixed flexor and extensor spasticity; that is, co-contraction. The original pure pattern of extensor spasticity with a relative inhibition of all flexor activity has become modified in order to make standing and walking possible. With the original total extensor pattern the child could neither stand or walk. He would fall backwards and not be able to flex and lift one lower limb to transfer his body weight forward.

The deformities which may result from the functional use of the abnormal patterns are the following:

(1) A kyphosis of the dorsal spine.

(2) A lordosis of the lumbar spine (Fig. 52).

(3) Subluxation or dislocation of one or both hips due to adduction of the thighs and insufficient development of the hip joints, resulting from late standing.

(4) Adduction and inward rotation of the legs, with flexor deformities of hips and knees, resulting in the typical scissor posture.

(5) An equinovarus or equinovalgus deformity of the feet.

Before deciding on an operation to bring the heels to the ground in these children, it is important to be certain in the individual case how much of a total flexor pattern is overlaid and hidden by extensor spasticity. In some children even a tendon Achilles lengthening operation may rob the child not only of extensor spasticity but also of sufficient extensor tone for standing. It may tip the scales towards total collapse into flexion.

Personality traits of the spastic group

The severely spastic child, both the quadriplegic and the more involved diplegic child, is very insecure. He is unable to move effectively, or to adjust himself to changes of posture, especially when he is moved quickly when handled by his mother: for instance when being washed, dressed, picked up, fed and so on. He cannot right himself when left in an uncomfortable position, and cannot maintain or regain balance. He is therefore in constant fear of falling if not sufficiently supported. He will often remain immature and dependent, clinging to his mother and reluctant to venture out into any independent activity. Often, the quadriplegic child cannot express himself with speech, gesture or movement. Eventually, therefore, he tends to protect himself from change, becomes withdrawn and passive and does not react to stimulation from the environment, as he knows from experience that he cannot respond adequately and that any attempt to do so usually results in failure and frustration.

Spastic hemiplegia

The aetiology of spastic hemiplegia is varied. In the newborn, prolonged labour, prematurity and birth asphyxia may all play their part. In early infancy and childhood, acute hemiplegia may be caused by convulsions or infections, such as meningitis or encephalitis (Tizard 1961). Children with hemiplegia due to causes acting before the age of about five years might still come within the definition of cerebral palsy, while after this time they approximate more and more to the picture of adult hemiplegia. In childhood the right side is more commonly involved, which Perlstein (1954) and Churchill (1968) ascribed to the more frequent left occipital position of the baby at birth. The early clinical picture has already been described, and should not be difficult to recognise. It is therefore surprising that hemiplegic infants still come to treatment relatively late, when the condition is usually well-established and mother and child both accept and are habituated to it. This is regrettable as there seems to be general agreement that early treatment gives far better and quicker results (Ellis and Culloty 1961, Skatvedt 1961, Köng 1962, 1965, 1966). Furthermore, once hemiplegia has become established and the child has achieved total orientation towards the normal side, it is one of the most difficult and challenging conditions to treat. The child can manage with the normal side and is reluctant to have anything to do with the hemiplegic side, preferring to look away from and disregard it. This is accentuated by the well-known frequent association of infantile hemiplegia with perceptual disturbances, such as impaired proprioception and especially, stereognosis. These disturbances may not necessarily be due to direct brain damage but are more frequently due to lack of experience, and can therefore often be greatly improved by early treatment. As stated before, the child may not appear very spastic initially; in fact, the affected side may be floppy in an acute case of hemiplegia. The child's motor development in general will be delayed, with late establishment of balance in sitting, standing and walking. He will show a tendency to fall towards the involved side, as he lacks both the balance reactions of the trunk and the parachute reaction of the arm on the affected side.

The child will gradually orient himself more towards the sound side, and fear, combined with lack of balance, will produce increased spasticity of the affected side (the result of associated reactions). He will prefer, in an emergency, to fall towards the sound side because he can then protect his head and face. In due course righting and equilibrium reactions will become hyperactive on the sound side in order to compensate for their absence on the affected side. At first the hemiplegic baby progresses along the floor in prone, turning his head away from the affected side and dragging along the hemiplegic arm and leg. He will first turn from supine to prone over the affected side by pushing himself off with the normal arm, and has difficulty in initiating turning over towards the normal side because of the retraction of the shoulder on the affected side (Fig. 53). While sitting, the whole of the affected side will be retracted (Fig. 54). This tendency to neglect the affected side will often be reinforced by the way the inexperienced mother handles her baby. He will not learn to crawl on hands and knees, but prefers to bottom-shuffle, that is, progress along on

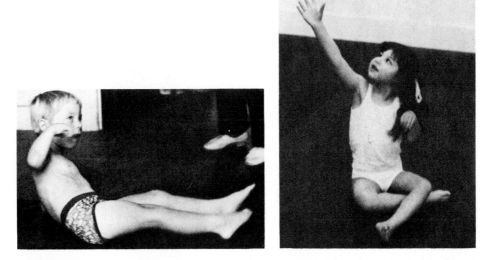

Fig. 53 (*left*). Child with right-sided hemiplegia sitting up by pushing with left arm. Note inward rotation of spastic right leg.

Fig. 54 (*right*). Child with left-sided hemiplegia sitting with weight on normal right hip with retraction of affected side. Reaching out with normal arm, there is strong association reaction in left arm.

his seat, pulling himself along with the sound arm and dragging the affected side along (Robson 1970, Robson and Mac Keith 1971). He will only learn to sit up and stand up with the help of the sound side, and the establishment of equilibrium in standing and walking will be somewhat delayed.

In standing, he will support his weight mainly on the sound leg. At first the affected leg will remain abducted with hardly any weight on it. It will appear to be 'weak' rather than spastic, and the child will tend to collapse if made to bear weight on it, because leg and foot are still mobile and he has therefore insufficient extensor tone to support his weight as long as his heel is on the ground and his knee is flexed and mobile. This difficulty can best be observed when the child attempts to walk downstairs. He cannot do this in the normal way, that is, by stepping down with alternating use of his legs, but has to use the affected side for stepping down, while bearing his weight on the flexed sound leg. At this stage he can usually put his heel on the ground quite easily. Because of the abduction pattern of the whole lower limb at this stage, his foot shows eversion rather than inversion, although his toes are already stiff in plantar flexion and will 'claw'.

In standing, the child is unable to transfer his weight onto his heel when tilted backwards (Fig. 55): if the child manages to raise and flex the spastic leg, it will flex at all joints, hip, knee and ankle. The leg may even abduct, which shows that the pattern of extensor spasticity hides a total flexion-abduction pattern of the spastic leg, with dorsiflexion of the ankle. This proves that the anterior tibial muscles are not weak but cannot act selectively within the total spastic extensor pattern of the leg, whereas in the flexion-abduction pattern the ankle is flexed and cannot be selectively plantiflexed. The same picture also shows the associated reaction of the spastic arm when effort is made to use the spastic leg. Some children may develop

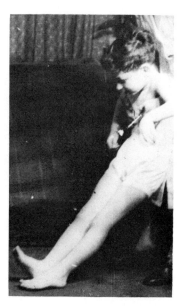

Fig. 55. Child with left-sided hemiplegia showing reaction to being tipped backward. Normal weight transfer onto heel is prevented by extensor spasticity in spastic left leg, with apparent weakness of tibialis anticus by reciprocal tonic inhibition through spastic triceps surae.

some additional distal athetosis around the seventh or eighth year.

As the child learns to walk, the leg and foot will gradually stiffen as he will have take his weight, at least momentarily, on the affected limb. He can only support his weight on the affected leg with the help of extensor spasticity, which is produced by the pressure of the ball of the foot against the ground. This means, however, that he has to walk on his toes. Extensor spasticity now gradually increases, and in many cases a pattern of inversion and plantar flexion of the ankle develops in addition to the 'clawing' of the toes.

In standing and walking, the child hyperextends his knee as there is insufficient extension of the hip joint for the transfer of body weight forward over the foot. To allow him to put his heel to the ground, his pelvis is kept rotated backwards on the affected side and his hip is held in some degree of flexion. He develops a pattern of walking very similar to his pattern of moving along the floor in the sitting position, dragging the affected side behind. At the same time, flexor spasticity of the upper limb increases, largely as the result of associated reactions; the forearm pulls up in walking and even more so in running. Associated reactions result from efforts of the sound side, *i.e.* the exclusive use of the sound hand and over-activity of the sound leg, and also from lack of balance and difficulty in raising the affected leg in walking. The opening of the fingers of the affected hand, for example, becomes increasingly difficult and possible only with a flexed wrist.

A hemiplegic child may in time develop the following contractures and deformities:

(1) Flexor deformities of elbow and wrist with pronation of the forearm and ulnar deviation of the wrist.

(2) Adduction of the thumb.

(3) Scoliosis of the spine. This is due to the spastic contraction of the side flexors of the trunk on the affected side. It will produce a pelvic tilt, as the pelvis will be drawn up on the affected side. The shoulder will be pulled down and this may be aggravated by shortening of the affected leg, owing to disturbances of growth through disuse or trophic impairment.

(4) An equinovarus or equinovalgus of the ankle, with shortening of the Achilles tendon.

The ataxic child

Pure ataxia in cerebral palsy is very rare, and early on is not readily recognised as it cannot be differentiated from the 'floppy infant'. The differential diagnosis of the 'floppy infant' is extremely difficult, especially with respect to the differentiation from infants with hypotonia due to genetically determined malformations of the central nervous system. Some guidance may be provided by the family history, or a lack of abnormal events during pregnancy and labour. In most cases of cerebral palsy this initial hypotonia will change; the child will subsequently develop athetosis (with or without intermittent spasms) or spasticity, or not infrequently an ataxic diplegia with spasticity, as described by Ingram (1954, 1964). The child who remains floppy will usually show a more or less severe degree of mental retardation. The differential diagnosis and classification of the floppy infant has been discussed by Lesny (1960) and Dubowitz (1969), and a good summary and informative article has been written by Sanner (1971).

A separate group of ataxias has been delimited by Hagberg and Lundberg (1969) and Hagberg *et al.* (1972), who described the 'dysequilibrium syndrome' characterised by a markedly defective postural function resulting in disturbed equilibrium, the distribution of which affects the trunk and legs, while arms and hands function normally. This condition develops after an initial period of muscular hypotonia. Hagberg also observed associated spasticity of the lower extremities in some of his cases. Thus it seems that the differential diagnosis of early hypotonia and cerebral palsy rests on careful history-taking, but certainty of diagnosis can only be obtained by following the further development of these children. Most cases of ataxic cerebral palsy are due to brain injury and are of a mixed character, the common factor in all ataxias being a persistently low postural tone combined with disturbed reciprocal innervation with lack of co-contraction, which makes sustained control against gravity and movement impossible or very difficult. Holmes (personal communication), when demonstrating a patient with disseminated sclerosis and marked ataxia, showed the importance of controlled reciprocal innervation for skilled and directed mobility. He demonstrated this with the finger-nose test. The patient began flexing one arm and the biceps contracted, while the triceps relaxed completely by near-reciprocal 'inhibition'. The patient tried to correct the 'overshooting', and, in doing so, reversed the movement. Now the triceps contracted and the biceps quickly relaxed again. Repetition of this process explains the resulting 'intention tremor' which is due to the patient's attempts to correct the failing reciprocal interaction. Holmes demonstrated this neatly in an experiment in which he tied an elastic band around the forearm of the patient, holding one end of it. The patient was now able to do the same movement smoothly and without difficulty, as the elastic band took over control which the relaxing antagonist could not exert.

Lesigang (1973, 1976) and Haidvogl (1979) have described a special type of 'floppy infant' characterised by a dislike of the prone position. They develop good head and trunk control, with normal use of hands and arms, after some delay. The most characteristic feature, however, is their unwillingness to assume the standing position. They flex their legs in the air as if 'sitting in the air'. They have a good prognosis, both physically and mentally, with normal final development. As Haidvogl stresses, this syndrome is also described by Hagberg *et al.* (1972) among his so-called 'dyskinetic group', but it is not specially differentiated. It is also among the group described by Robson (1970) and Robson and Mac Keith (1971) under the term 'bottom shufflers'. It is perhaps unfortunate to describe this group under the term 'dissociation syndrome', as dissociation of motor development, also described by Illingworth (1960), with a scatter in the various fields of motor development, is characteristic for every baby with brain injury.

The motor development of ataxic children is usually delayed, with the attainment of milestones occurring much later than normal. Their movements are jerky and uncontrolled, and their head and trunk control remains poor, so they are often unable to sit before the age of 15 or 18 months. Sitting, even then, is somewhat unstable, and only possible in the more severe cases by the adoption of a wide sitting base with flexed and widely abducted legs. However, if, the legs at that time develop spasticity, sitting up may be delayed further still by extensor spasticity of the legs. Standing and walking may be very delayed, for two or three years or longer, and the child will be very unstable and tend to fall a great deal. Fine hand and finger movements and the manipulation of objects are clumsy, and there may be an added intention tremor. Frequently, there is the added difficulty of lack of eye movements independent from head movements, and these children are therefore unable to follow an object or use their eyes to control their hand movements. Speech is often delayed and slurred, characteristically with an open mouth and considerable dribbling (drooling).

Personality traits of the ataxic child

The fear of losing balance and the child's awareness of his slow and inadequate mechanism of postural adjustment make him move slowly and carefully. He will limit the range of movement patterns voluntarily, or move only those he can control and feel safe with. He may keep his eyes fixed on the floor or on a non-moving object and dare not move his head. He may therefore hold himself stiffly, walking with a wide gait for safety. He often cannot stand still, since he adjusts his balance in standing by making steps rather than by postural adjustment of the head and trunk. The typical stance is shown in Fig. 56*a-d*. Acquired forms of ataxia, not strictly belonging to the cerebral palsies but occurring in childhood, are due to meningitis, encephalitis as a result of virus infections, and—not infrequently—due to road accidents. These are usually mixed cases with spasticity or rigidity. The typical instability of trunk is shown in sitting (Fig. 56*e*).

The athetoid group

Many aetiological factors contribute to this very varied group. One of the most important factors used to be blood incompatability, especially the Rh-factor. The identification of Rhesus iso-immunisation and subsequently its prevention and treatment may have produced a significant fall in the number of cerebral-palsied children from 2 per thousand to about 1.5 per thousand, with a decline in the number of athetoid children (Hagberg 1969).

All athetoid children show an unsteady and fluctuating type of postural tone. In the pure cases, basic postural tone is below normal and the amplitude of the fluctuation varies widely in the individual child, depending on the severity of the condition, and the degree of stimulation and effort. These children lack a sustained postural tone and ability to fixate, due to impaired reciprocal innervation. They lack proximal co-contraction and are therefore unable to maintain a stable position against gravity. Their inability to control their movements and give postural fixation to the moving part interferes with the performance of manual skills. They are in many ways the counterpart of the spastic child in whom permanent hypertonus and exaggerated co-contraction produce an exaggerated static attitude at the expense of mobility. The athetoid child, unless his condition is complicated by spasticity, lacks grading of antagonistic and synergistic activity during a movement. Contraction of one group of muscles leads to an almost complete inhibition of the antagonists; what is lacking is the dovetailing of agonists, antagonists and synergists, so necessary for

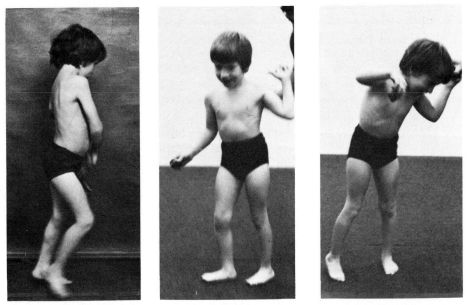

| Fig. 56a | Fig. 56b | Fig. 56c |

Fig. 56. Spastic diplegic with ataxia: (*a*) walking; (*b*) and (*c*) showing unstable balance in standing supported; (*d*) unable to balance; (*e*) unstable trunk in sitting. (For *d* and *e* see facing page).

strength and control of any movement. Movements are therefore jerky, uncontrolled and extreme in range, with poor control of the mid-ranges.

Head control is poor and the upper limbs are usually more involved than the lower limbs. In pure cases the lower extremities are usually primitive rather than abnormal. Because of the lack of co-contraction and the extreme ranges of movement combined with low postural tone, there is hypermobility of all joints with a tendency to subluxation, especially of the mandibles, shoulder and hip joints and the fingers.

The distribution of the condition is usually very asymmetrical, head control is often poor, very often associated with disturbances of eye control, speech and hearing. These children frequently have feeding difficulties, with open mouths and constant dribbling. A child with a markedly asymmetric condition may have strong intermittent spasms to one side, resulting in rotatory spasms and a marked intermittent torticollis.

Breathing is usually very abnormal, and vocalising, especially at request, difficult, whereas vocalising under emotional stress is often surprisingly good. In many children articulation is not too bad, but voice production is poor in nearly all of them, especially with respect to sustained sound. Normalising of the body musculature tone with treatment often has a surprising effect on speech and breathing.

Personality traits of the athetoid group

All patients of this group appear to be unstable and somewhat unpredictable in their response to stimulation. They seem to have a low threshold to excitation when in a state of hypertonus and a high threshold with delayed response when hypotonic.

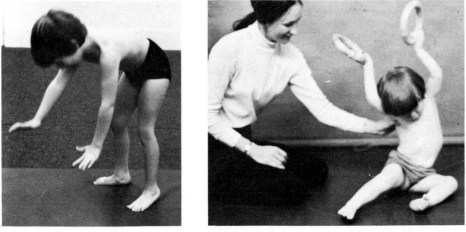

Fig. 56d	**Fig. 56e**

They show quick and extreme changes from one state to another, both physically and emotionally, and are quick to laugh and cry uncontrollably. They have sudden outbursts of temper, while otherwise gay and outgoing, laugh easily and cry with abandon.

Types of involuntary movement

All these types of involuntary movement are reinforced during any attempt at volitional activity, when the patient tries to co-ordinate a purposeful movement against the background of unstable postural tone, in spite of the interference by tonic reflexes. They can be usefully grouped as in Fig. 57.

These groups are not sharply divided, but show many transitional and mixed types. Group I and III are divided only by their response to stimulation. A baby who starts in group III may change later on to group I, or more rarely to group II. Group

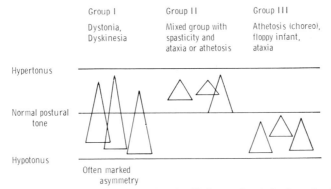

Fig. 57. The athetoid group of cerebral palsy classified according to basic postural tone and response to stimulation. Each triangle represents a single case; the baseline represents the type of tonus at rest, and the amplitude represents the basic tone under stimulation.

II also includes occasional mixtures of ataxia (Ingram's ataxic diplegia).

Fluctuations of postural tone are sudden and manifest themselves in some of the involuntary movements seen in all cases of the athetoid group. In the individual case we may see the following types of involuntary movements:

(*a*) *Intermittent tonic spasms.* These are predictable in pattern and are largely dependent on a change of the position of the head; that is, they are due to the influence of the tonic labyrinthine and neck reflexes. They may fix the child temporarily in certain extreme postures of total flexion or extension (tonic labyrinthine influence), or in asymmetrical postures of extension of the limbs on the face side and flexion of the limbs on the occiput side (asymmetrical tonic neck reflex influence). There may be a mixture of both in the individual case.

(*b*) *Mobile spasms* (Wilson and Walshe 1914/15) These involve the limbs in alternating movements of flexion and extension, pronation and supination, etc. They are often rhythmic in nature. Examples are the 'athetoid dance' (spinal stepping reflexes) and pawing of the ground with one foot.

(*c*) *Fleeting localised contractions.* These affect muscles or muscle groups anywhere in the body, and if they are strong and affect many muscle groups they may produce grotesque and exaggerated postures and movement, such as grimacing of the face, and bizarre attitudes and movements of hands and fingers. Their patterns of co-ordination are quite unpredictable and the law of reciprocal innervation is in abeyance in this type of involuntary movement (Wilson 1920, 1925). These postures and movements defy attempts at imitation by a normal person. If these localised muscular contractions are weaker and more limited they may show themselves only in minor localised twitches.

Most children in the athetoid group have quadriplegia, in which the head and upper parts are more involved than the lower parts. A few hemiplegic cases are seen among those with some distal athetosis; this appears usually around or after the sixth or seventh year. More rarely one sees children with pure hemi-athetosis.

In athetoid quadriplegia, postural tone is usually low during the first two to three years. Their postural patterns resemble those of a premature child rather than those of a fullterm baby. Righting reactions may not develop for many years and may remain defective even in later life. Head control is absent or very poor, the child being unable to raise his head in supine or prone lying. In the supine position he is unable to initiate sitting up or to turn over to prone or side lying. The baby cannot tolerate lying in prone, as he is unable to raise his head, extend his spine and hips or use his arms for support. He cannot get up on his hands and knees and is unable to crawl. He may therefore spend the first years of his life lying in supine or sitting propped up. He commonly holds his head to one side, usually the right, and cannot move it into midline or maintain it there. When pulled to sitting the child's head lags excessively. He is unable to lift it off the support and in fact it is pulled backwards (Fig. 58).

As the child grows older and starts to react more to environmental stimulation, postural tone develops and becomes stronger. He now suddenly stiffens with increasing frequency, and in the supine and sitting positions throws his head backwards with extension of hips and spine (Ingram 1954, Polani 1959). The patterns of these intermittent extensor spasms are often the only motor patterns in the supine position of which the child makes voluntary use for moving himself backwards along the floor. This he does by bending his legs and pushing his feet, which are less affected, against the floor. At this stage the asymmetrical tonic neck response activity is usually very strong and affects not only the upper limbs but the whole of the trunk (Fig. 59). The resulting asymmetrical postural pattern produces a scoliosis with tilting of the pelvis, which is sometimes followed by a subluxation or dislocation of one hip (usually the left).

He usually retains a primitive flexion-abduction pattern of the lower limbs unless there is additional spasticity, in which case the legs will show a typical extension-adduction pattern. Sitting up is delayed and very difficult because of extensor resistance and poor head control. He can only achieve this by pulling himself up with the help of the hip flexor. The retention of the abduction-flexion pattern makes sitting on the floor possible later on, as it gives the child a wide sitting base. Sitting is also made possible through some equilibrium reaction of the less-affected hips and legs. Although he may not be able to pull himself to sitting, since he cannot lift his head or use his arms, when pulled to sitting he may assist in the movement by strong active flexion of the hips.

Although he is unable to control his head when being pulled to sitting, once he has reached the sitting position the child may be able to hold his head up and keep his spine erect, but his head will be turned to one side. In sitting he may learn to use one hand, usually the left, turning his head to the right and using the pattern of the asymmetrical tonic neck reflex for grasping. His grasp is usually weak, however, and he releases objects too easily and cannot hold on to a support. This is quite different from the tonic grasp of the spastic child, who cannot open his hands but holds on tightly to an object placed into his palm, and which in fact he cannot release.

Although the athetoid child may be able to sit on the floor with extended and abducted legs, he cannot sit unsupported on a chair as this requires additional flexion of the knees. This flexion would produce a total flexion pattern of the body, resulting in the patient's falling forwards and down, especially if he could not use his arms and

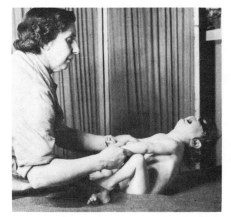

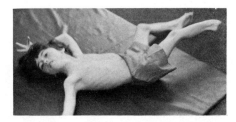

Fig. 59 (*above*). Athetoid quadriplegic child in supine. Note asymmetry and retraction of head, neck and shoulders.

Fig. 58 (*left*). Athetoid quadriplegic child pulled to sitting.

hands for support (Fig. 60a). If he raises his head in sitting, a total extensor pattern results and he falls backwards (Fig. 60b), showing a primitive Moro reflex on falling into extension (Fig. 60c).

If the lower limbs are not too badly affected the child will learn to roll over to his side and prone lying, initiating the movement with his legs. From the prone position, though he is unable to raise his head or to support himself on his arms, he will manage to get himself to a kneeling position by first pulling his legs into total flexion under his body. He can then raise his head and use his arms for support in extension, making use of the symmetrical tonic neck reflex. He can thus move into kneel-sitting, but he cannot alternately extend and flex his legs and is only able to hop along the floor in this position. Kneeling on all fours and normal crawling is impossible.

Standing and walking will depend on the relative normality of the child's legs and on the degree of head control and equilibrium which he can develop. He usually cannot use his hands to hold onto a support, to pull himself up to standing or to hold on when walking. Extensor spasms tend to make him fall backwards, and both this and the asymmetrical distribution of postural tone interfere with balance. The constant fluctuation of postural tone make for insufficient support tonus. It may take him years to stand for any length of time and many children whose lower limbs are badly involved may not stand or walk at all. When they are made to stand, the legs are in total extension-adduction pattern and may even cross. These children stand high on their toes, their neck and shoulders are retracted, and they tend to fall backwards. If they flex one leg to make a step, they may collapse in full flexion.

Other children whose lower limbs remain mobile and retain abduction, not only in sitting but also in standing, will learn to stand and even to walk. However, they use a primitive pattern of stepping, lifting their legs too high. The abduction pattern of the lower limbs, together with dorsiflexion and eversion of the feet, will give them a sufficient walking base. They walk with hyperextended hips and knees and lean the trunk and shoulder girdle backwards to avoid collapse in flexion, in this way reinforcing extensor tonus (Fig. 61) sufficiently to maintain standing.

Many athetoid children seem to have some element of ataxia. This applies especially to those with a basically low postural tone. The ataxic element, however, is

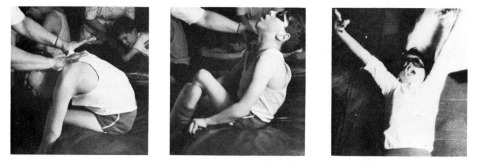

Fig. 60. Child with athetoid quadriplegia: (*a, left*) with head down he is pulled into flexion and (*b, centre*) with head up he falls backward; (*c, right*) Retention of primitive Moro reflex on falling into extension.

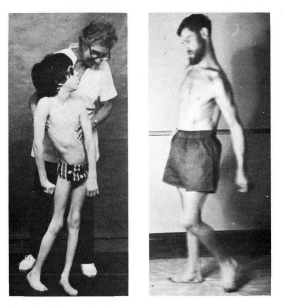

Fig. 61. Typical standing and walking patterns of athetoid quadriplegia.

difficult to differentiate from athetosis if involuntary movements are very marked. If athetosis is slight and distal in distribution, the ataxic element may be very clear. Athetosis, with its lack of a sustained postural tone, insufficiency of co-contraction and lack of a proper grading of 'reciprocal innervation', demonstrates a type of postural tone that is very similar to that seen in ataxia.

The athetoid child is not likely to develop deformities as long as postural tone is generally low and he is hypermobile, and he has, in fact, too many patterns. However, because of his hypermobility he may show a tendency towards subluxation or dislocation of the mandible, shoulder and hip joints, and of the fingers.

The mixed cases in this group, that is the athetoid with spasticity or the dystonic child with strong intermittent increases of postural tone, may develop the following contractures or deformities:

(1) A scoliosis of kyphoscoliosis, often associated with deformities of the chest wall.
(2) Flexor deformities of elbows and wrists, the wrists showing severe flexion, with extended and 'weak' fingers.
(3) Flexor deformities of hips and knees, with equinovarus or equinovaglus of the ankles.
(4) Dislocation of one or both hips, usually the left.

CHAPTER 8

The Early Recognition of Cerebral Palsy

Clearly, this chapter might logically have come at the beginning of the book, but it is only when one has a thorough understanding of what one is looking for that one can begin to identify cerebral palsy cases early.

The first signs are usually those of an arrest or retardation, with the retention of the primitive and total synergies of earliest childhood. However, abnormal signs will appear, such as hypertonus, spasticity or the intermittent spasms found in the athetoid group (Crothers and Paine 1959, Paine 1960, 1964, Paine and Oppé 1966). The evolution of the pathological signs, like the development of normal motor development, also takes a cephalo-caudal direction. Therefore, whereas the normal baby develops extension against gravity in prone, and flexion against gravity in supine, the abnormal patterns of hypertonus will lead to a spread of extensor tone in supine and flexor tone in prone, pulling the child in the direction of gravity. How quickly this develops will depend on the severity of the condition and the distribution of the abnormalities in the individual case. Although by definition the lesion is stationary, the symptomatology is not, appearing gradually and often progressing over many years. First symptoms may appear immediately following, or even during, a stormy perinatal period, but these cases present no particular diagnostic problem. In other instances there may have been some abnormalities during the pregnancy, followed by a relatively normal perinatal period of varying length, after which symptoms appear. These cases may present diagnostic problems.

There is great difficulty in differentiating the pathology from permissible signs of deviation from normal development. Illingworth (1960, 1962) rightly stresses these difficulties and describes babies with unusual symptomatology who subsequently develop normally. He stresses the importance of repeated examination and assessing the baby's rate of development, a point also emphasised by Hart *et al.* (1978). This is especially so in babies under four months, particularly with a history of prematurity. There is no doubt that if one treats babies of this age and does not take into account the deviations from normal, one will be treating a large number of normal babies. It is often very difficult to establish a definite diagnosis of cerebral palsy before the end of the fourth month and even then it may be impossible to say what type of cerebral palsy the child is likely to develop, and what the final outcome will be in terms of distribution and severity of the pathology. It must be remembered that, not infrequently, signs of a deviation in motor development may be observed without any prognostic significance. Lesigang (1976), for instance, has observed that babies nursed on their abdomen may be beautifully extended in prone, with very early head control. However, they may not be able to raise their head in supine to initiate sitting up until they are nine months old. We have also observed this in abnormal babies who are treated almost exclusively in prone and who may be unable to sit up or are afraid to sit up even at the age of two or three years. Early recognition must therefore depend on routine development assessment at regular intervals. As Egan *et al.* (1969) have stressed, a developmental assessment should be just as much part of any examination of a baby as is listening to his heart. However, in a baby with suspected brain damage the intervals between seeing the baby should be short, and certainly not more than two or three weeks apart after the appearance of suspicious signs. It must be remembered that during the first year of a baby's life development is at its fastest and 'soft signs' may become 'hard signs' over a very short time. The early diagnosis rests to a large extent on the differentiation of primitive signs of delay from those of a pathological nature, which in the individual picture may show themselves side by side.*

Parents often bring their baby to the doctor because he has not reached the usual milestones at the accepted time; that is, usually around the eighth month when the baby should sit up, or even later. A thorough history-taking is then called for, followed by the *usual paediatric and neurological examination*. A history of one or more of the following is to be found in many of the children; abnormal birth, prematurity, asphyxia, anoxia, breech, prolonged labour, precipitate labour, a small-for-dates baby, twinning, multigravida mother, etc. The mother may have her nights disturbed by a fretful baby, or the nights may be undisturbed and the baby may have been too quiet and placid; both types of babies may also have feeding difficulties. Many mothers will state, either spontaneously or on questioning, that the baby could not be placed on his tummy, as he could neither raise the head nor turn it to one side. When examining the baby it should be kept in mind that the tests described here have been developed empirically in order not only to make an early diagnosis but also, and perhaps more importantly, to give indications of the child's needs in treatment. They aim at assessing the baby's handicap in terms of the abnormal signs, and also at explaining in what way they interfere with the baby's 'principal' and functional abilities. In this way a rational treatment and management programme can be planned. An assessment like this also has a predictive value and may show what will become of the child if he be allowed to use the developing abnormal motor patterns for purposive activity.

So far, little is known about the relationship between certain prenatal and perinatal events and specific types of cerebral palsy, although there are some connections indicated by epidemiological research. Thus, prematurity is not infrequently associated with spastic diplegia (Brandt and Westergaardt-Nielsen 1958) and Rh and other blood incompatibilities with athetoid types of cerebral palsy. In the latter cases, transitory hypotonia, sooner or later followed by marked fluctuations of postural tone on stimulation or effort, may indicate a future dystonic type of cerebral palsy.

While taking the history and establishing some contact with the mother and her baby, observation of each of them may give valuable information. As Ingram (1962) said, "There is a danger that attention paid to reflexes in infants may lead to a neglect

---

*Primitive signs can be defined as patterns of activity belonging to very early stages of a normal, fullterm baby's postnatal life, signs which were present once, but should have become modified and have disappeared. Pathological signs are motor patterns not seen at any stage of a normal baby's postnatal development.

of observations of their spontaneous behaviour from which so much more information of clinical value can be obtained''. Both the way the mother holds and supports the baby and the way the baby moves may indicate a stiff or floppy infant. One can watch whether the baby moves his toes, opens his hands, and how much support the mother gives to the head or trunk while the baby sits in her lap. Observation can also indicate whether the baby follows his mother with eyes and head, whether he reacts to sound while his mother holds his attention. Here the tests and techniques worked out by Sheridan (1968, 1973) are of immense value for testing vision and hearing. One should also note whether the mother talks to her baby while handling him; thus any examination already begins with a period of observation with the baby in the lap of his mother.

After this preliminary observation the baby is then tested in the ways described below. As already stressed, the traditional paediatric and neurological examination should not be omitted. Some typical results of specific testing techniques are described and exemplified by one or two examples of babies with cerebral palsy. It is useful to keep in mind that a normal baby develops his control of gravity in a cephalo-caudal direction, and likewise in the child with cerebral palsy the pathology also develops from the head down, and the baby is prevented from any movement in supine or prone, except the stereotyped patterns described below.

Tests in supine

This is usually the position of maximal extensor hypertonus. The fully developed case is shown in a child with severe spastic quadriplegia at 13 months (Fig. 62). The baby is fully extended, with head and shoulder retraction. The spine is straight, the legs adducted and extended at hips, knees and ankles. The arms are flexed at the elbows and the hands fisted. The baby is totally helpless, cannot lift his head, flex his hips and spine, and therefore cannot sit up. Retraction of the shoulders makes turning to the side or into prone impossible. The arms cannot be moved forwards, nor touch the body, and the hands cannot open and grasp an object.

The baby in Figure 63 was referred to the physician because of suspected cerebral palsy at six months old. He was brought to the clinic because his mother

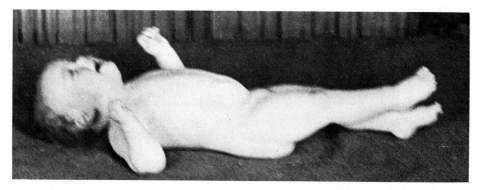

Fig. 62. Spastic quadriplegic at 13 months, showing full picture of extension spasticity in supine.

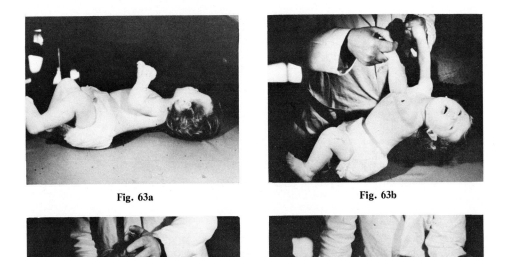

Fig. 63a

Fig. 63b

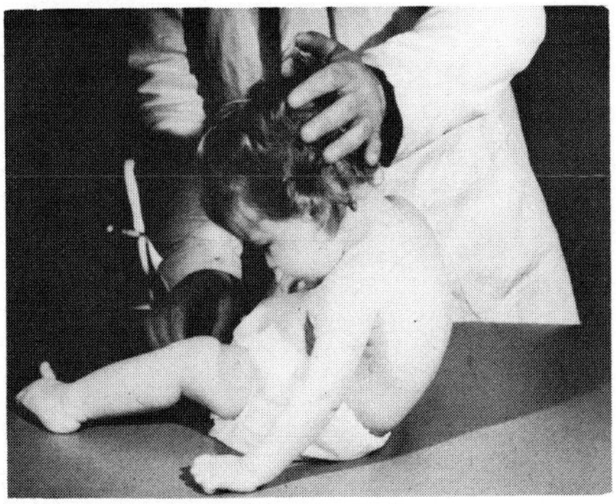

Fig. 63c

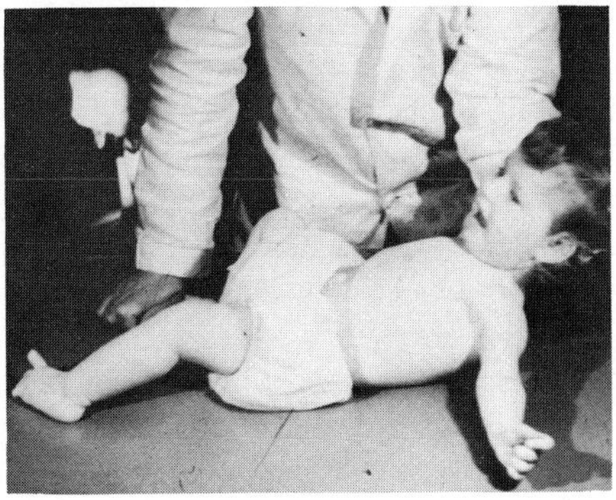

Fig. 63d

Fig. 63. Six-month-old suspected of having cerebral palsy (see text): (*a*) showing head retraction; (*b*) head lag on pulling to sitting; (*c*) pushed to sitting showing compensatory kyphosis instead of hip flexion; and (*d*) primitive Moro with asymmetry.

noted a delay in his reaching the usual milestones. He shows a typical mixture of possible abnormality and primitive motor patterns*. The possible pathology is seen in the head retraction (Fig. 63*a*), while the attitude of flexion of trunk and limbs is characteristic of a baby of two or three months. Whether or not this flexion denotes retardation depends on the changeability of the attitude under observation. The normal baby of three months opens his hands and fingers and brings them to his mouth and chest. He also kicks and has individual movements of ankles and toes. If, however, he cannot move in this way and cannot bring his hands to his mouth, and shows immobility or poverty of movements or asymmetry (for instance in kicking with one leg only), this would denote abnormality rather than retardation. Here the only definite sign of possible pathology is the retraction of the head and upper spine. The question is whether this is the first sign of developing extensor hyperactivity which will in time extend cephalo-caudally. The head retraction at this age is not necessarily

*The photographs in this chapter are of various infants, to show all stages in the development of spastic quadriplegia.

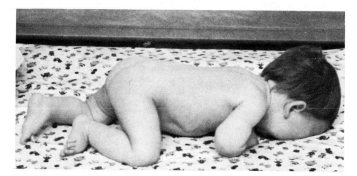

Fig. 64. Six-month-old in prone showing pathological head position in midline and primitive flexion.

abnormal, as babies at this stage frequently practise extension by throwing the head back and arching the spine in preparation for sitting and, later, standing. However, they put their feet against the ground and push their bottom up while doing this. The retraction of head and neck here is suspicious, as it does not fit into this usual pattern. By making various sounds and using large objects, the child's ability to hear and to follow an object with eyes and head is tested.

The baby is now pulled into sitting by his arms and shows considerable head lag throughout the range of lifting (Fig. 63b), that is, a lack of head control not seen even in the normal newborn. If next he is pushed into sitting by the examiner (Fig. 63c) he indicates clear pathology. Characteristically, he now shows a reversal of the usual response of a normal baby. The hips seem to resist flexion and the child can only come forward by a compensatory kyphosis. This shows that in time extensor spasticity will proceed and eventually involve the lower extremities. This suspicion is confirmed by the fact that in response to this handling the extended leg has turned inwards and is adducted, with the foot plantiflexed in a definite plantar extensor response. More important still, this abnormal reaction gives a clear indication of the future, showing that the child, if he is able to sit later on, will sit in the typical manner of many spastic children; that is, with insufficient hip flexion compensated by a dorsal kyphosis.

If the head is now allowed to drop back and is caught by the examiner the baby shows a primitive Moro reaction which is combined, however, with a further sign of pathology — an asymmetry, with left leg extended and adducted with plantiflexion, the other leg still in a primitive attitude of flexion-adduction, typical of spastic quadriplegia (Fig. 63d). If the head is rotated to one side, retraction of the shoulders may prevent the body from following.

Tests in prone

This is usually the position of maximal flexor hypertonus. The baby here again looks like a baby at a younger stage of development, with a complete flexion pattern. However, the head is maintained in midline, and cannot be raised, nor even be turned to one side (Fig. 64). The shoulders are unduly protracted with the arms adducted, and they sometimes get trapped under the body. The lack of head control both in

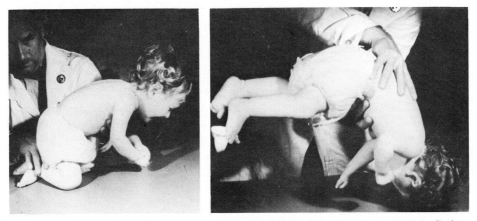

Fig. 65. Six-month-old (*a, left*) lifted by shoulders showing insufficient head control and primitive flexion, and (*b, right*) lifted by pelvis showing asymmetry, right side more severely involved than left.

supine and prone proves that this is not due to immaturity of the righting mechanism of the head (as is the case in normal babies, who can raise the head in prone long before raising it in supine). If the baby is lifted by the shoulders (Fig. 65*a*) the arms will flex, preventing the baby from being able to push himself up by supporting himself on his extended arms. If the baby is now lifted by the pelvis (Fig. 65*b*) the legs may extend and adduct, resisting flexion (due to symmetrical tonic neck reflex).

Held in the Landau position the baby is unable to raise his head, the arms are flexed and the legs sometimes extended and adducted (probably as the result of a symmetrical tonic neck reflex). If the baby is then tilted head first towards a surface, the flexed arms will prevent the normal parachute reaction.

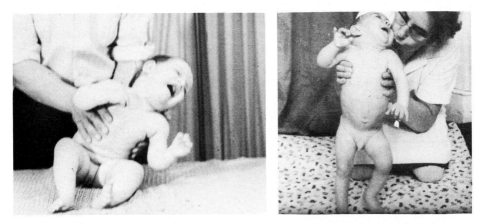

Fig. 66 (*left*). Infant displaying total lack of balance, trunk stability and parachute reaction.
Fig. 67 (*right*). Seven-month-old with severe spastic quadriplegia; head thrown back in pathological asymmetrical tonic neck response.

Tests in sitting

The baby is unable to sit. Flexor hypertonus of the arms prevents the parachute reactions forwards and sideways (Fig. 66). The head is poorly controlled.

Standing and vertical suspension (head down)

In standing with support, the baby's legs are extended and abducted and the feet are extended (Fig. 67) at a time when the normal baby usually pulls his legs up in flexion. In vertical suspension the baby is held by both legs (see Fig. 10, page 13) and normally if the one leg is then released it will fall into flexion (Collis 1947, 1954, Vojta 1974). In cerebral palsy, however, extensor spasticity will prevent this reaction. This finding adds little to the information gained by the other tests and is an expression of severe early spasticity only, and not, as stated by Collis, a sign of mental retardation. Assessing the baby's reactions in this way (that is, relating his reactions in supine, prone, sitting, Landau and standing to each other and not in isolation) is therefore valuable not only in arriving at a more certain diagnosis early, but also in giving a good idea of the future development and the aims of treatment.

Discussion

To sum up: this baby will develop into a typical spastic quadriplegic. Head control is poor, both in supine and prone, and the baby is very asymmetrical, the left side more severely involved than the right. He lacks extension in prone against gravity, and trunk control. These are the main features, indicating not only diagnosis but also the main objects to be attained by early treatment.

The early signs of athetoid quadriplegia

This is a whole group with very varying aetiology, and will present early on either as a 'floppy infant' or a rigid infant. Great difficulty may be experienced in the early recognition of the hypotonic type of cerebral palsy (the so-called 'floppy infant') and in deciding during this phase what the final type of cerebral palsy will be. It may even be very difficult to decide whether it is a cerebral palsy at all, or whether the hypotonia is of a congenital myogenic type (Ingram 1954, 1964, Dubowitz 1969, Robson 1978). In the baby with cerebral palsy, hypotonia is a transitory symptom followed sooner or later by an unsteady and fluctuating type of postural tone (dystonia) characteristic of the athetoid group, with disturbance of reciprocal innervation and lack of co-contraction. Hypotonia may also be followed by the development of a spastic or plastic hypertonus. The hypotonic phase is usually seen in the very young baby who does not as yet try to move and, if persistent, is often associated with mental retardation. It may also persist in babies who subsequently develop cerebellar ataxia. These do not strictly belong to the cerebral palsy grouping. It also develops into a special type of ataxia described by Hagberg *et al.* (1972) as 'dysequilibrium syndrome' or, in association with spasticity, as mixed ataxic-spastic diplegia described by Ingram (1964). These are discussed on page 58. During the hypotonic phase there is little resistance or response to passive stretch of muscles and therefore an increased range of passive movement. The child shows little discomfort if placed in what would normally be an uncomfortable position and he has little urge to move or to right himself. Typically, however, increase of postural tone, even to hypertonus (though intermittent and at first fleeting in nature), can be produced by adequate stimulation and in response to handling.

During the first few months the baby usually lies on his back with one or both legs widely abducted and flexed at hips and knees and with the thighs resting on the supporting surface. The feet are dorsiflexed and everted and can easily be made to touch the anterior aspect of the leg, a primitive pattern present in the normal baby during the first few weeks of life. The arms are retracted at the shoulders and flexed at the elbows (also a primitive normal baby pattern).

As the condition develops, the baby may show a strong and intermittent asymmetrical tonic neck reflex, affecting not only the arms (which would be primitive) but also the trunk, as evidenced here by a scoliosis and marked asymmetry of trunk and limbs. The legs continue to show predominantly exaggerated primitive postures, with the right leg in total flexion, outward rotation, and with marked 'clawing' of the toes, the left leg in a primitive extension pattern with some inversion at the ankle (Fig. 68a). If the baby is pulled to sitting (Fig. 68b) he shows marked head lag, although with the head in midline the asymmetry disappears. When he is pushed to sitting (Fig. 68c) the arms and shoulders persistently pull back even after he has moved forwards past the vertical position (Fig. 68d). The more usual response is a slump forward into total flexion when the trunk is moved beyond the vertical (Fig. 69a). The baby also has difficulty turning the head from side to side when following an

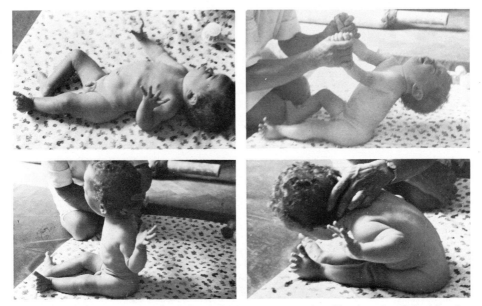

Fig. 68. Athetoid baby at 5½ months: (*a, top left*) asymmetry, retraction of head, neck and shoulders, legs in more primitive position; (*b, top right*) pulled to sitting (with the head in midline the asymmetry has disappeared); (*c, bottom left*) pushed to sitting, shoulders and arms press backward (again, with head in midline the asymmetry has disappeared); (*d, bottom right*) resistance persists when pushed forward in flexion.

object. He is unable to turn from supine to either side or over to prone because of the shoulder retraction.

When placed in prone he may not be able to raise his head, but may just turn it to one side (Fig. 69b). The arms remain by the sides in flexion or caught under the body, the legs spread out into flexion abduction to such an extent that the groin sometimes touches the supporting surface. Some babies, however, may be able to raise their head and support themselves on their arms and they are more symmetrical than in supine.

At later stages, as the child starts to react to stimulation and to being handled and moved about, postural tone develops, but not normally. He may then develop intermittent fluctuations of postural tone of varying amplitude. These will tend towards exaggerated extension in supine, when the child responds to handling by throwing himself backwards in a total extension pattern, called 'dystonic attacks' by Ingram (1955) and 'opisthotonic attacks' by Polani (1959) (Fig. 69c). These attacks may also occur in supported sitting, when the child's head drops back, and may be associated with the retention of a primitive Moro reflex. In ventral decubitus the baby is unable to raise the head and the Landau reaction is absent (Fig. 69d).

The early recognition of this type of cerebral palsy and its differentiation from

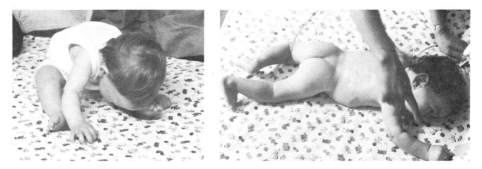

Fig. 69a   Fig. 69b

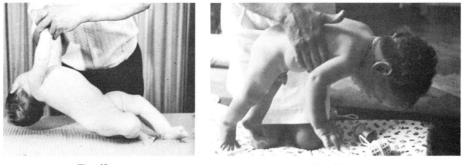

Fig. 69c   Fig. 69d

Fig. 69. Six-month-old baby with athetoid quadriplegia: (*a*) unable to sit upright, the baby slumps forward (this is a more usual reaction than that in Fig. 68*d*): (*b*) in prone, there is more primitive flexion and insufficient head control; (*c*) a dystonic attack; (*d*) absent Landau response.

other causes of hypotonia rests on the interpretation of the child's response to handling which aims at the early discovery of any potential hypertonic reactions to stimulation. Handling in supine and supported sitting may provoke excessive extensor activity—the influence of the tonic labyrinthine reflex—and also, at times, responses characteristic of the asymmetrical tonic neck reflex. Flexor hyperactivity in prone may be demonstrated by raising the baby up by his shoulders. His arms will pull upwards in flexion against gravity, indicating that the child's inability to raise his head may not only be due to the general hypotonic condition but to hyperactivity of the flexors. A valuable diagnostic sign has been described by Lesny (1960); namely, that if the baby is held in vertical suspension with his feet above the ground and moved down towards the support he may pull up his legs in flexion against gravity (Fig. 70). In standing he is unable to extend the legs.

The early signs of hemiplegia

The early diagnosis of hemiplegia is usually not difficult because of the early appearance of asymmetry in posture and movement. The face is usually turned away from the hemiplegic side, but the head may be laterally pulled towards it. There is often some retraction of the shoulder on the side of the affected arm. Intitially, however, spasticity is mild and the hand is still open, with some flexion of the fingers and some adduction of the thumb (Fig. 71a). The leg may initially be flexed at all joints and abducted, with persistent marked clawing of the toes. The baby will not pass through any important symmetrical stage of development and therefore does not use both hands in midline. He also does not reach out and grasp with the involved hand. In prone he cannot support himself well on the affected arm (Fig. 71b). Kicking of the affected leg is less lively than normal. In sitting, the affected shoulder

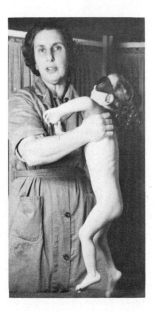

Fig. 70. Early pattern of athetoid quadriplegia; unable to maintain standing because of primitive flexion in lower extremities.

will show some retraction. Later on the arm and hand are used only when absolutely necessary, and gradually the child will orient himself more and more towards the functionally sound side (Fig. 71c).

In prone when lifted by the hips the spastic leg extends stiffly and the arm is in a flexion-pronation pattern due to associated reactions (Fig. 71d). The parachute reaction is absent in the hemiplegic arm (Fig. 71e) and when pulled to sitting the hemiplegic leg extends stiffly (Fig. 72).

A comprehensive study of the hemiplegic infant and child, and of their treatment has been written by Treml (1975).

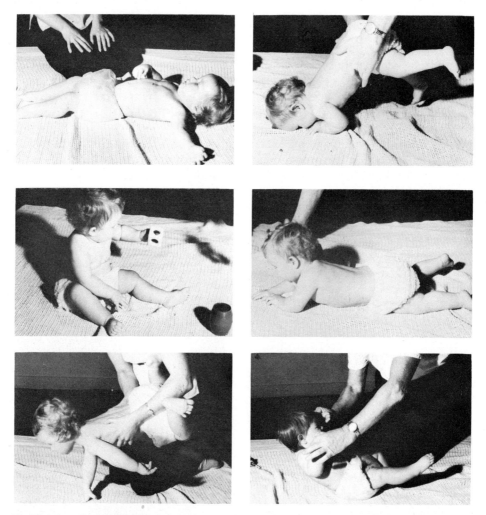

Fig. 71. Infant with left-sided hemiplegia: (*a, top left*) using normal arm in supine; (*b, top right*) in prone; (*c, centre left*) sitting, using normal right arm; (*d, centre right*) lifted by hips; (*e, bottom left*) absent parachute reaction in spastic left arm; hemiplegic leg extends when pulled to sitting.

Fig. 72 (*bottom right*). Infant with right-sided hemiplegia; when pulled to sitting, right leg extends stiffly.

CHAPTER 9

The Treatment of Cerebral Palsy

Some neurophysiological facts

The treatment of children suffering from cerebral palsy has been developed purely empirically, based on the analysis of the various types and their development, and rests on two principles:

(1) The inhibition or suppression of the abnormal tonic reflex activity which is responsible for the patterns of hypertonus.

(2) The 'facilitation' of the normal, higher integrated righting and equilibrium reactions in their proper development sequence, with a progression towards skilled activities (Semans 1967, Manning 1972, 1976).

We call the second principle 'facilitation' because experience of treating these children has shown that the righting and equilibrium reactions are potentially present in most cases. They occur either spontaneously or can be 'activated' easily once the tonic reflexes are successfully inhibited. These normal reactions are obtained as automatic responses of the infant and child to specific techniques of handling (Bobath and Bobath 1964, Manning (now Bryce) 1976).

It must be stressed that the treatment has largely evolved and been developed purely empirically during the last thirty-five years. However, it has achieved more normal motor function than the forms of treatment which disregard the neurological nature of the child's handicap. There is a need to explain the empirically observed facts of treatment, if at all possible, in terms of established neurophysiological knowledge.

The concept developed here should be considered as no more than a working hypothesis to explain the observed facts. However, it must be remembered that, as Denny Brown (1950, 1962a, b,) has stressed, we know a great deal about the structure of the central nervous system but our knowledge of its function is largely speculative. He stated, "Knowledge of the anatomy of the brain has always been considerably more extensive than that of its physiology. From the beginning there has been a constant tendency to identify anatomic structure with categorical functions and to claim for the resultant scheme the status of a physiological system. It is unfortunately true that the 'functions' attributed to the motor regions of the frontal cortex, the pyramidal tract and various extrapyramidal motor structures in our most authoritative textbooks of neurology and neurophysiology to-day bear critical analysis little better than the 'faculties' plotted by the phrenologists" (Denny-Brown 1950).

Perhaps some remarks made by Ritchie Russell in an address to the Royal Society of Medicine (1958) may be of relevance. Speaking on the 'Physiology of Memory', he said, "There is first the apparently fundamental tendency for nerve cells to repeat patterns of activity, so that all reactions have a strong tendency to form arrangements which are repeated whenever possible, and around which more elaborate responses are built. The tendency to repeat seems to be one of the most powerful features of all nervous activity."

Later on, Ritche Russell adds "The activity of the mature CNS usually falls into well-worn patterns which have formed during years of development. These furrows of habit become first ruts to guide and then chains which control our responses to a greater or lesser extent. These bonds of habit affect simple motor responses very strongly so that our very movements assume a unique character." This tendency to form bonds of habitual motor activity finds expression in the similarity of man's fundamental activities, like sitting up, sitting, getting up, standing and walking.

From birth onwards we are activated by powerful stimuli which come to us from the outside world through our exteroceptors, especially the distance receptors, our eyes and ears. They are the initiators of our motor responses which are subsequently guided and controlled throughout their course by the feedback from muscles, tendons and joints, that is, from our proprioceptors. In the guidance of movements initiated by the exteroceptors, the proprioceptors are therefore of great importance (Walshe 1948). Twitchell (1954) rightly stresses the importance of sensory factors in the performance of movements and functional skills.

The mature and intact central nervous system is able to absorb a large amount of afferent inflow, and reacts to it with variable responses, adapting to the changing conditions of the environment. The intact nervous system has at its command a great variety of discrete and selective motor responses and can adjust posture and equilibrium accordingly.

The central nervous system of the child with cerebral palsy is less competent to deal with the afferent inflow, although there may be no impairment of the sensory and perceptual system. Although the child may retain the ability for unitary and integrated reponse, this response is more often stereotyped by being short-circuited into the synaptic chains of a few typical patterns of abnormal reflex activity. The child's motor responses mainly consist of a few spinal and tonic reflexes, although one or other of the more highly integrated righting and equilibrium reactions may occur. These form the primary abnormal sensorimotor patterns which in their interplay determine the child's motor output, and which the child changes and adapts in the performance of functional skills (Held 1965). The dominance of these primary reflexes results in abnormal secondary or compensatory patterns which, if unchecked, lead to contractures and deformities. The fundamental handicap of a child with cerebral palsy is therefore not one of input, unless this is also affected, but one of elaboration within the central nervous system and output. Any treatment, therefore, which approaches the problem purely from the sensory or input aspect, using special types of sensory stimulation, such as brushing (Goff 1969, 1972), vibration or ice (Kabat 1952, 1958, 1959, Hagbarth and Eklund 1968) misses the fundamental problem. To express this idea another way, expecting a child with cerebral palsy to react to these types of sensory stimulation with a more normal output is no more realistic than expecting to teach a cat to walk on two legs. The patterns of activity are just not available to the child, as they are overlaid and inhibited by abnormal reflex activity. One can, of course, reduce hypertonus by techniques of relaxation, that is, by understimulation. However, this will not help the child; on the contrary it will very often make the child more sensitive and more likely to react abnormally under normal conditions of stimulation.

The short-circuit patterns of hypertonus act more or less permanently in the spastic or rigid child, and intermittently in many of the athetoid, especially dystonic, group of children in whom spasms interfere with voluntary activity. In the child with true athetosis or ataxia, hypotonia and lack of sustained reciprocal innervation make postural control and skilled activity impossible.

Sooner or later in the growing child the abnormal sensorimotor patterns of the hypertonic state become firmly established in his central nervous system. It is important to attempt to prevent this by early treatment and management. The afferent inflow is shunted into the few synaptic chains established by the dominance of spinal and brainstem reflexes, with the addition of perhaps one or the other of the automatic reactions of the midbrain and cortical centres. In milder cases the abnormal patterns are modified by voluntary and compensatory activity, but the underlying primary abnormal patterns, although changed by compensatory and abnormal motor activity, can often still be inferred.

The central nervous system and integration of motor function

The idea of the short-circuiting of the sensory input in cerebral palsy is illustrated by a simplified sketch of the central nervous system (Fig. 73) with its four main levels of integration of motor functions, as studied by Magnus (1924), Sherrington (1939) and Schaltenbrand (1925, 1927) and many others. These levels of integration have been derived from animal experiments and therefore cannot be simply translated in terms of human neurophysiology. However, in spite of this limitation it is probable that the hierachical scheme of motor levels is still valid, but it should be thought of as a gross simplification of a very complex interplay of functional, rather than anatomical, levels.

Level 1 (the spinal animal)

Section of the central nervous system at this level produces the 'spinal animal' showing the various spinal reflexes studied by Sherrington, among them the flexor

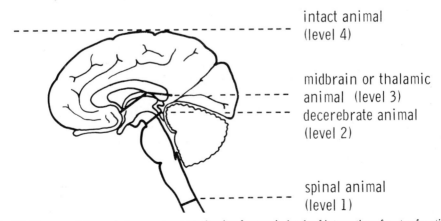

intact animal
(level 4)

midbrain or thalamic
animal (level 3)
decerebrate animal
(level 2)

spinal animal
(level 1)

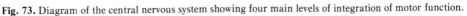

Fig. 73. Diagram of the central nervous system showing four main levels of integration of motor function.

79

withdrawal reflex, the extensor thrust, and the crossed extension reflex. These are pure phasic reflexes, or reflexes or movement. They are, however, functionally very useful patterns for swimming and progression along the ground. They should be considered as the basic building stone which higher centres adapt and modify for more complex functional activities in the course of phylogenetic development, especially the necessary activity of resisting gravity. It is noteworthy that Sherrington devoted much time and effort to the study of CNS activity at this level. He rightly stressed that the integrative action of the central nervous system was qualitatively the same at every level, the main difference between higher and lower levels being a matter of complexity and quantity rather than quality. It was therefore easier to study the laws of nervous activity at the spinal level, and then look at the modifications imposed upon these at higher levels. He showed the 'inhibition' at the spinal level was a primitive factor affecting movement in total patterns only, as evidenced by spinal reciprocal inhibition. He also showed that this inhibition was an active process exerted by the central nervous system and that it was in fact 'central' inhibition. He stressed its importance as a co-ordinating factor in posture and movement (Sherrington 1913). In cerebral palsy, it can be shown that underlying the hypertonic patterns, the result of release from higher inhibitory control, there are mass movement patterns of the spinal type which in their turn are inhibited by the presence of spasticity and its patterns.

Level 2 (the decerebrate animal)

Section at this level just below the red nucleus produces the 'decerebrate animal' studied by Magnus (1926), Rademaker (1935) and Sherrington (1947). After the shock of decerebration has worn off, the animal becomes rigid because of a strong increase in postural tone in all muscles, with a predominance of hypertonus in the antigravity muscles. Sherrington called this state 'decerebrate rigidity'. This is unfortunate, as this type of hypertonus is quite different from the 'rigidity' of Parkinsonism, and is better termed 'maximal spasticty'. Our understanding of spasticity, as for instance the activity of the gamma system, has been based on studies on decerebrate animals. At this level the phasic reflexes of the spinal cord are modified; reciprocal 'inhibition' become reciprocal 'innervation', which allows the animal to stand but only in an abnormal manner, due to exaggerated postural tone and 'co-contraction'. The animal can remain static in this fixed position, but once unbalanced cannot restore itself to this position. This is exactly what 'spasticity' is; namely, a state of exaggerated fixation caused by hypertonus and excessive co-contraction. The tonic reflexes responsible for maintaining this abnormal posture against gravity are the result of a philogenetically older state of postural control. One may look upon spasticity as nature's first clumsy attempt to solve the problem of postural control against gravity. What should be re-emphasised here is that the central nervous system is always concerned with patterns of activity rather than the activity of single muscles.

Level 3 (the midbrain or thalamic animal)

Magnus (1926), in his experiments on cats and dogs, found little difference whether the thalamus was removed or remained intact; the important factor was the production of a state of 'decortication'. In this state we have for the first time 'reactions' rather than reflexes; that is, automatic responses adaptable to a change of condition. Unfortunately they are described as 'reflexes' in the literature (Schaltenbrand 1925, Magnus 1926, Rademaker 1931), but it is essential to realise that at these higher levels the central nervous system acquires its most fundamental and important capacity, that of adaptation to changing circumstances. Thus the outstanding quality of the higher CNS activity is its plasticity, that is, its ability to learn; and perhaps one should also add the 'gift of forgetting', the ability of forming temporary and constantly changing chains of synaptic corrections in response to the many and various demands of the environment. At this level postural control is fairly normal and the distribution of postural tone adjustable, and the animal is able to assume and maintain a normal position. It is of some interest, however, that the righting function is often exaggerated and obligatory in these animals, reminiscent of some hyperkinetic children with brain injury.

Level 4 (the intact animal)

Postural control and tone are perfect. The righting reactions in the adult animal are fully integrated, with perfect equilibrium reactions. The latter probably result from a close and harmonious interaction between the sensorimotor cortex, the thalamic and subthalamic structures, and the cerebello-pontine-cerebral systems.

In children with cerebral palsy we rarely find a total disruption of the neuraxis comparable to any one of the experimentally produced levels of integration mentioned above. The lesions are either extensive and scattered, or they are more localised and do not produce a complete interruption of the neuraxis at any one level. It is therefore unusual to see in children the clear-cut clinical picture which has been described in experimental animals. Furthermore, one has to remember that experimental studies on animals at different stages of phylogenetic development have shown somewhat different results from the same lesion. Tower (1935, 1940), for instance, has shown that the same lesion produces different motor disturbances in monkeys and apes, and that the latter had more lasting and severe deficits. Wilson (1920) described states of partial and total decerebrate rigidity in man and the occurrence of intermittent decerebration with 'tonic fits'. Byers (1938) described children with cerebral palsy and grouped them according to a partial or total decerebration syndrome.

As stressed before, in the child with cerebral palsy the afferent inflow is short-circuited mainly into the synaptic channels of tonic reflex activity, that is, level 2 of the scheme described above. However, in most cases apart from the very severe ones, both levels 3 and 4 may modify the clinical picture to some extent. Hence a child with a moderate degree of hypertonus may be able to move without any great increase in postural tone so long as he moves within the tolerance of the damaged central nervous system. For example, many athetoid children show one or other of the righting and equilibrium reactions, or they may compensate with fairly normal, or even normal, reactions of the non-involved parts for shortcomings of the affected parts. However, these movements are interfered with by the intermittent action of tonic reflexes, producing transient abnormal postures similar to those seen in the spastic child. The picture may be further complicated by involuntary movements which are probably due to the disturbed feedback of the sensorimotor cortex with thalamic or subthalamic structures.

A problem in treatment is implied by this interpretation of the child's handicap; one may either accept that the short-circuit created by the lesion is unalterable, or else attempt to change it. If we can accept the former on the grounds that destroyed brain-matter cannot be replaced and is not capable of recovery, then it follows that the only reasonable way of helping the child is to teach him to make the best use of his abnormal motor patterns for voluntary movements. We have to support the child in developing compensatory abnormal patterns and help him to adapt them as best he can for functional use. This means accepting the necessity of splinting and bracing to protect the child from contractures and deformities, and using surgical measures to alleviate them once they are established.

The interpretation presented above does help to explain the rationale of treatment which aims at inhibiting the abnormal patterns of hypertonus and facilitating the higher integrated postural reactions, which are the prerequisite of functional activity against a background of normal postural tone and equilibrium. Below I shall attempt to answer the question of whether or not this is possible, by considering the 'rule of shunting' stated by Magnus (1924).*

'The rule of shunting' and its rôle in treatment

Before discussing the rule, it may be helpful to outline its history. Sherrington (1913) found that in a spinal frog one and the same stimulus applied within the same receptive field of a particular reflex could in certain circumstances have directly opposite results. For instance, stimulation of the toe area of the frog's extended leg produced a flexor withdrawal reflex. However, if after repeated stimulation the leg flexed and remained flexed for a while, the same stimulus produced an extensor thrust ('shunting'). Sherrington called this phenomenon "reflex reversal". He found this phenomenon of reflex reversal surprising and asked Magnus to investigate it. Magnus first established by a number of experiments that reflex reversal was a common pheno-menon. He also found that for a specific shunt to result, *i.e.* for a stimulus to follow a specific pathway within the CNS, the proximal joints were of major impor-tance; for instance, if a leg was flexed at the hip but extended at knee and foot, the result would more likely be flexion than extension of the leg, and vice versa. Searching the scientific literature for similar observations, he found the writings of van Uexkuell (1905), who had studied the response to stimulation of primitive organisms, such as the starfish. He had excised one of the five 'legs' of the starfish, together with its connection with the very simple central nervous system, and placed it in a box, the central part being in the box, with the foot hanging down through a hole (Fig. 75). The whole box was fixed to a stand in such a way that it could be rotated through 180 degrees. The tip of the hanging leg was then stimulated and the leg rose up against gravity, the upper muscles contracting and the muscles on the underside

*It must be stressed, however, that the ideas developed here only serve to explain the empirically established facts, and the concept developed here, although speculative, is certainly useful as a working hypothesis and serves to explain the clinically observed facts.

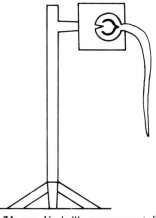

Fig. 74. van Uexkell's arrangement for demonstrating effect of elongation of muscles on reflex responses.

relaxing by reciprocal inhibition. He repeated the experiment with the box turned through 180 degrees and again the leg was raised, due this time to contraction of the previously inhibited muscle groups.

From these and similar observations on the behaviour of simple organisms, van Uexkuell stipulated the shunting rule as it applied to simple reflex activity and the reactions of primitive organisms. He stated that the results of any stimulation can be predicted by looking at the state of the body musculature; the actively contracted muscles will be in a state of central inhibition, while the elongated antagonists will receive excitatory outflow from their central nervous system.

If we look again at Sherrington's original experiment we find that the fact of simple 'reflex reversal' can be explained by this rule of van Uexkuell. However, Magnus extended the rule, giving it a significance far beyond the mere explanation of primitive or reflex activity. He expressed it as a general rule of normal motor response in highly developed organisms, including man.

He stated that "at any moment during a movement or a postural change the CNS mirrors, or reflects faithfully, the state of the body musculature." Expressed another way, he was stating that at any moment during a movement or postural change the distribution of excitatory and inhibitory processess within the CNS reflects the state of the body musculature. It is therefore the body musculature which guides and directs the CNS. It is the body musculature which controls the opening and closing of synaptic connections within the CNS and determines the subsequent outflow. This is only another way of expressing the fact, already mentioned, that the exteroceptors, especially eyes and ears, initiate an activity, but that the proprioceptors guide and determine its course (Walshe 1921).

If we accept this rule, it is clear that we can influence the state of the central nervous system from the periphery through sensory channels by changing the abnormal postural patterns of the child; by handling the child and directing his active responses away from the undesirable spastic patterns, that is, away from the channels of abnormal reflex activity, we can hope to stop the outflow of excitation into

TABLE II

An example of the competing patterns of the lower extremities

Extension	Flexion
Extension of the hip	Flexion of the hip
Extension of the knee	Flexion of the knee
Adduction of the leg	Abduction of the leg
Inward rotation of the leg	Outward rotation of the leg
Plantiflexion of the ankle	Dorsiflexion of the ankle

hypertonic patterns. At the same time we are opening up the channels of higher and more normal muscular activity. The treatment principles thus consist of two factors:
(1) Inhibition of the outflow into the synaptic chains of the abnormal reflex patterns responsible for hypertonus, that is, its 'reflex inhibition'.
(2) 'Facilitation' of the higher integrated normal postural reactions, in this way normalising postural tone and activating the righting and equilibrium reactions, with progression towards normal functional ability.

In the child with cerebral palsy, it is possible to apply the rule of shunting in its simple form as stated by van Uexkuell, since we are dealing to a large extent with released abnormal *reflex* activity. The two main patterns of the lower extremities of a spastic or athetoid child may serve as an example of its application. However, it should be kept in mind that when treating a child, the whole condition must be taken into consideration; treatment of the lower extremities only may result in increased hypertonus of the rest of the involved parts as a result of 'associated reactions'. In treatment, then, the therapist will pay special attention to the whole body in order to prevent this. The two competing patterns of the hypertonic leg (Milani-Comparetti 1964) are shown in Table II.

The chart shows that according to van Uexkuell's rule it should be easy to change the spastic extension pattern into one of total flexion and vice versa. This is indeed the case, as seen both by a child's own effort and in some treatments. For instance, the hemiplegic child has either a total extension pattern of the leg or a total flexion pattern. It has already been shown that within the total extension pattern he cannot flex the ankle, whereas he cannot plantiflex it within the total flexion pattern. Furthermore, many diplegic and quadriplegic spastic children cannot flex their knees in prone without the hips pushing upwards in flexion and the leg abducting. The hips will also flex if the child in supine tries to flex the spastic leg. On the other hand, many mixed athetoid children show a total flexion-abduction picture, unless they have some additional spasticity. Based on this fact of two competing total patterns in the spastic child, Fay (1948, 1954, 1955, 1958) developed a treatment which aimed at overcoming spasticity with the help of the spinal reflexes, using his 'unlocking of reflexes' technique. These techniques were developed further by the 'patterning' of Doman *et al.* (1960), and later Vojta (1974), where approach to treatment was based on a combination of the techniques of Kabat (1958) and Fay.

However, neither of the total patterns (see Table II) will lead to normal standing and walking. For functional activity both the spastic extension patterns *and* the total flexion patterns have to be modified, and elements of one pattern must be combined with elements of the other. This is beautifully demonstrated in the developing infant, where the flexion and extension patterns—seen in the kicking and walking of the normal infant—are gradually modified. At four months the baby can already flex his knees in prone independently and with relative extension of the hip.

For the purpose of combining elements of both total patterns, various reflex-inhibiting patterns have been devised. The child is handled in such a way as to combine flexion of hips and knees with adduction of the leg. In prone, in preparation for standing, the lower extremities are moved into outward rotation and abduction, combined with extension of the hips and knees. Whilst doing this, pressure is applied against the feet. This builds up sufficient extensor tone for standing, while at the same time inhibiting extensor spasticity. An athetoid child with a total flexion-abduction pattern of the leg may be treated with a pattern of adduction and extension of the legs, and the mother must be discouraged from carrying the child on her hip with flexed and abducted legs.

These reflex-inhibiting patterns must not be looked upon as static postures, but as phases of movement away from the total patterns. It is also important to appreciate that these patterns by themselves achieve nothing; the child will learn nothing from being moved passively. What is of decisive importance is his reaction to these movements away from his established pathological patterns, and his active adaptation to these reflex-inhibiting movements. It is therefore important in the individual case to find the limit of his tolerance to being handled and to discover at what point in being handled he begins to react abnormally. At this point treatment has to step in to stop the hypertonus with its abnormal patterns from asserting itself, and gradually to increase his tolerance to stimulation and handling. Hypertonus and its patterns are release phenomena; treatment aims at restoring inhibitory control to the child. This can only be done by giving the child the necessity and the possibility of developing his own inhibitory control. In this process of gradually building up inhibitory control one is really imitating nature, repeating phylogenetically what already occurs in a normal baby, since the child with cerebral palsy can be considered as phylogenetically primitive. In the individual case, inhibition of abnormal reflex activity and facilitation of normal righting and equilibrium reactions and movements may either follow each other or be used alternately, or simultaneously. Whichever way inhibition and facilitation are combined, it is essential that the child be given a chance to move actively. The reflex inhibiting movements are initiated from certain key points of control, predominantly from the head and neck or other proximal parts of the body, such as the shoulder girdle, spine and pelvis. These are the parts of the body where both normal and abnormal motor activity originate. This is evidenced by the fact that both the tonic labyrinthine and tonic neck reflexes produce abnormal distribution of hypertonus and that the normal neck righting and labyrinthine righting reactions on the head initiate normal postural control. Normal postural control against gravity starts with head control and proceeds in a cephalo-caudal direction, and modification of limb movements proceeds from proximal to distal. The degree and distribution of hypertonus of the extremities therefore can be successfully controlled and influenced from these proximal key-points, and by changing the child's position at key-points only, it is possible to control inhibition of abnormal postural movement patterns. The child is left free to move his limbs actively while the therapist controls the key-points, preventing any influx of hypertonus and deterioration of movement. This allows for the combination of simultaneous inhibition and facilitation. By carefully choosing and constantly changing the key-points of control, one can obtain a whole sequence of active automatic movements without interference by abnormal patterns.

In more severe cases, as in older children with a spastic or plastic hypertonus, techniques of inhibition are still predominantly used in treatment for as long as is necessary to reduce postural tone sufficiently to allow for facilitation of active movement responses. However, even head righting and equilibrium reactions have to be facilitated as soon as possible. In all other cases, especially babies and very young children with moderate spasticity or athetosis, facilitation techniques are used simultaneously with inhibition. Babies do not usually show appreciable degrees of spasticity or athetosis, and techniques of facilitation can be used effectively to obtain normal responses, only using inhibition to stop interference by abnormal reactions. Abnormal motor patterns, except in severe cases, have not yet become established; in fact, these babies have usually moved very little. With early treatment, the development and habituation of faulty movement patterns can be prevented and normal patterns be given a chance to develop. By facilitating righting and equilibrium reactions, entire sequences of movement, such as rolling over, sitting up, sitting unsupported, standing up and even walking, may be achieved. Righting reactions can usually be developed in all but the most severe cases, but it may be impossible to obtain the full orchestra of equilibrium reactions, especially in standing and walking.

For an explanation of the effect of facilitation we return again to Russell (1958). He cites evidence from neurophysiological studies which show that synaptic transmission along certain chains can be greatly facilitated by previous activity along the same connection. Therefore, there is evidence of a neuronal mechanism which favours repetition, and this is true for every level of the central nervous system.

He continues, "It is equally evident, that this complicated neuronal activity is extremely sensitive to outside (afferent) influences. Apparently the neuronal pool can be alerted to make responses which take priority over spontaneous activity, so that if a certain response has in the past followed a certain experience there is every likelihood that it will be repeated in the future to the same stimulus, until it acquires a remarkable degree of constancy and automaticity." We may add that this is especially so if the newly facilitated reactions belong to phylogenetically and ontogenetically established patterns, like the righting and equilibrium reactions.

When applying this to treatment principles, it means that the permanent carry-over of treatment depends largely on the extent to which the higher reactions can be facilitated and their synaptic chains firmly established by repetition. These higher reactions permanently modify and keep in check the released abnormal reflexes, thus keeping postural tone adequate and steady. This also underlines the importance of early recognition and management, before abnormal patterns have become established.

With this approach to the treatment and management of the child, the degree of success that can be reached in any particular case depends largely on the potential of the child's damaged brain; that is, to what extent higher integrated motor responses, overlaid by abnormal activity, can be evoked and established in treatment.

In some of the hypotonic ataxia and athetoid children, and in children with intermittent spasms, in whom postural tone after successful inhibition is low and who lack sustained reciprocal innervation and co-contraction, it may be necessary to increase tone and to regulate reciprocal interaction. Special additional techniques of proprioceptive and tactile stimulation, such as pressure, weight-bearing and resistance, serve this purpose. They have to be used with great care, otherwise these techniques of strong stimulation may easily produce hypertonic reactions, so the child's reactions have to be watched carefully. The neurophysiological rationale underlying these techniques is the recruiting of gamma-activity by repeated tactile and proprioceptive stimulation, increasing postural tone to the necessary extent and regulating reciprocal interaction for fixation of proximal points and controlled and selective movement distally.

NOTES

REFERENCES

Abercrombie, M. L. J. (1960) 'Perception and eye movements; some speculations on disorders in cerebral palsy.' *Cerebral Palsy Bulletin,* **2,** 142-148.

—— (1968) 'Some notes on spatial disability: movement, intelligence quotient and attentiveness.' *Developmental Medicine and Child Neurology,* **10,** 206-213.

André-Thomas (1940) *Equilibre et Equilibration.* Paris: Masson.

—— Autgaerden, S. (1966) *Locomotion from Pre- to Postnatal Life. Clinics In Developmental Medicine, No. 24.* London: S.I.M.P. with Heinemann; Philadelphia: Lippincott.

—— Chesni, Y., Saint-Anne Dargassies, S. (1960) *The Neurological Examination of the Infant. Little Club Clinics in Developmental Medicine, No. 1.* London: National Spastics Society.

—— Saint Anne Dargassies, S. (1952) *Etudes Neurologiques sur le Nouveau-Né et le Jeune Nourrison.* Paris: Masson et Oliver Perrin.

Bax, M. C. O. (1964) 'Terminology and classification of cerebral palsy.' *Developmental Medicine and Child Neurology,* **6,** 295-297.

Bazett, H. C., Penfield, W. G. (1922) 'A study of the Sherrington decerebrate animal in the chronic as well as the acute condition.' *Brain,* **45,** 185-265.

Beevor, C. E. (1903) 'The Croonian lectures on muscular movements and their representation in the central nervous system.' *British Medical Journal,* **1,** 1357-1360.

Bench, J., Collyer, Y., Langford, C., Toms, R. (1972) 'A comparison between the neonatal sound-evoked response and the head-drop (Moro) reflex.' *Developmental Medicine and Child Neurology,* **14,** 308-317.

Bobath, B. (1965) *Abnormal Postural Reflex Activity Caused by Brain Lesions.* London: Heinemann Medical.

—— (1967) 'The very early treatment of cerebral palsy.' *Developmental Medicine and Child Neurology,* **9,** 373-390.

—— (1968) *Abnorme Haltungsreflexe bei Gehirnschäden.* Stuttgart: Thieme.

—— (1969) 'The treatment of neuromuscular disorders by improving patterns of coordination.' *Physiotherapy,* **55,** 18-22.

—— (1971*a*) 'Motor development: Its effect on general development and application to the treatment of cerebral palsy.' *Physiotherapy,* **57,** 526-532.

—— (1971*b*) 'The effect of spasticity on adult hemiplegia and its treatment.' *Physiotherapy,* **57,** 456-458.

—— Bobath, K. (1975) *Motor Development in the Different Types of Cerebral Palsy.* London: Heinemann Medical.

Bobath, K. (1959*a*) 'The effect of treatment by reflex-inhibition and facilitation in cerebral palsy.' *Folia Psychiatrica, Neurologica et Neurochirurgica Neerlandica,* **62,** 448-457.

—— (1959*b*) 'The neuropathology of cerebral palsy and its importance in treatment and diagnosis.' *Cerebral Palsy Bulletin,* **1,** (8), 13-33.

—— (1960) 'The nature of the paresis in cerebral palsy.' *Report presented to the Second National Spastics Society Study Group, Oxford.*

—— (1962*a*) 'Two views on the tonic neck reflex.' *Developmental Medicine and Child Neurology,* **4,** 220, *(Letter.)*

—— (1962*b*) 'The neurophysiology of cerebral palsy.' *Pädiatrische Fortbildung Praxis,* **48.**

—— (1963) 'The prevention of mental retardation in patients with cerebral palsy.' *Acta Paedopsychiatrica.* **30,** 141-154.

—— (1966) *The Motor Deficit in Patients with Cerebral Palsy. Clinics in Developmental Medicine, No. 23.* London: S.I.M.P. with Heinemann; Philadelphia: Lippincott.

—— (1971*a*) 'The problem of spasticity in the treatment of patients with lesions of the upper motor neuron.' In: *Proceedings of the 6th International Congress of the World Federation for Physical Therapy, Amsterdam, 1970.* Assen: van Gorcum.

—— (1971*b*) 'Frühbehandlung und ihre methodischen Grundlagen.' In: Matthias, H. H., Bruester, H. T. (Eds.) *Spastisch Gelähmte Kinder.* Stuttgart: Thieme.

—— (1971*c*) 'The normal postural reflex mechanism and its deviation in children with cerebral palsy.' *Physiotherapy,* **57,** 515-525.

—— Bobath, B. (1964) 'The facilitation of normal postural reactions and movements in the treatment of cerebral palsy.' *Physiotherapy,* **50,** 246-262.

Boyd, I. A., Meyers, R., Swinyard, C. A. (1964) *The Role of the Gamma-System in Movement and Posture.* New York: Association for the Aid of Crippled Children.

Brandt, S., Westergaard-Nielsen, V. (1958) 'Etiological factors in cerebral palsy and their correlation with various clinical entities.' *Danish Medical Bulletin,* **5,** 47-52.

89

Brimblecombe, F. S. W., Richards, M. P. M., Roberton, N. R. C. (1978) *Separation and Special Care Baby Units. Clinics in Developmental Medicine, No. 68.* London: S.I.M.P. with Heinemann; Philadelphia: Lippincott.
—— (1976) 'The management of spasticity in children.' Physiotherapy, **62**, 353-357.
Bühler, C. H. (1927) *Inventar der Verhaltungsweisen des Ersten Lebenjahrs.* Jena: Gustav Fischer.
—— (1935) *From Birth to Maturity.* London: Routledge & Kegan Paul.
—— Hetzer, H. (1928-32) *Kleinkindertests.* Leipzig: J. A. Barth.
Byers, R. K. (1938) 'Tonic reflexes in children.' *American Journal of Diseases of Children,* **55**, 696-742.
Churchill, J. A. (1968) 'A study of hemiplegic cerebral palsy.' Developmental Medicine and Child Neurology, **10**, 453-459.
Collis, E. (1947) *The Way of Life for the Handicapped Child; A New Approach to Cerebral Palsy.* London: Faber.
—— (1954) 'Some differential characteristics of cerebral motor defects in infancy.' *Archives of Disease in Childhood,* **29**, 113-122.
Crothers, B., Paine, R. S. (1959) *The National History of Cerebral Palsy.* London: O.U.P.
Denner, B., Cashdan, S. (1967) 'Sensory processing and the recognition of forms in nursery-school children.' *British Journal of Psychiatry,* **58**, 101-104.
Denny-Brown, D. (1950) 'Disintegration of motor functions resulting from cerebral lesions.' *Journal of Nervous and Mental Diseases,* **112**, 1-45.
—— (1962a) *The Basal Ganglia and their Relation to Disorders of Movement.* London: O.U.P.
—— (1962b) 'The midbrain and motor integration.' *Proceedings of the Royal Society of Medicine,* **55**, 527-538.
Doman, R. J., Spitz, E. B. Zucman, E., Delacato, C. H., Doman, G. (1960) 'Children with severe brain injuries: neurological organization in terms of mobility.' *Journal of the American Medical Association,* **174**, 257-262.
Dubowitz, V. (1969) *The Floppy Infant. Clinics in Developmental Medicine, No. 31.* London: S.I.M.P. with Heinemann; Philadelphia: Lippincott.
Egan, D. F., Illingworth, R. S., Mac Keith, R. C. (1969) *Developmental Screening 0-5 Years. Clinics in Developmental Medicine, No. 30.* London: S.I.M.P. with Heinemann; Philadelphia: Lippincott.
Ellis, E., Culloty, V. (1961) 'The treatment of young children.' In: *Hemiplegic Cerebral Palsy in Children and Adults. Little Club Clinics in Developmental Medicine No. 4.* London: Spastics Society with Heinemann Medical.
Fay, T. (1954) 'Use of pathological and unlocking reflexes in the rehabilitation of spastics.' *American Journal of Physical Medicine,* **33**, 347-352.
—— (1948) 'The neurophysiological aspects of cerebral palsy.' *Archives of Physical Medicine and Rehabilitation,* **29**, 327-334.
—— (1955) 'The origin of human movement.' *American Journal of Psychiatry,* **111**, 644-652.
—— (1958) 'Neuromuscular reflex therapy for spastic disorders.' *Journal of the Florida Medical Association,* **44**, 1234-1240.
Flehmig, I. (1970) 'Neurologische untersuchungen zur früherkennung zerebraler Bewegungsstörungen bei soggenannton Risikokindern.' *Materia Medica Nordmark,* **22**, 340-347.
—— (1975) (1975) *Die Denver Entwicklunsskalen.* Stuttgart: Thieme.
—— (1979) *Normale Entwicklung des Sauglings und Seine Abweichungen.* Stuttgart: Thieme.
Foley, J., Cookson, M., Zappella, M. (1964) 'The Placing and support reactions in cerebral palsy.' *Journal of Mental Deficiency Research,* **8**, 17-24.
Galant, S. (1917) *Der Rückgratreflex.* University Dissertation, Basel.
Gatev, V. (1972) 'Role of inhibition in the development of motor coordination in early childhood.' *Developmental Medicine and Child Neurology,* **14**, 336-341.
Gesell, A. (1938) 'The tonic neck reflex in the human infant.' *Journal of Pediatrics,* **13**, 455-464.
—— (1940) *The First Five Years of Life.* Vol. 1. New York: Harper.
—— Amatruda, C. S. (1945) *The Embryology of Behavior.* New York: Harper.
—— —— (1947) *Developmental Diagnosis, 2nd edn.* New York: Harper.
Goff, B. (1969) 'Appropriate afferent stimulation.' Physiotherapy, **55**, 9-17.
—— (1972) 'The application of recent advances in neurophysiology to Miss M. Rood's concept of neuromuscular facilitation.' Physiotherapy, **58**, 409-415.
Gooddy, W., MacKissock, W. (1951) 'The theory of cerebral localisation.' *Lancet,* **1**, 481-483.
Griffiths, R. (1954) *The Abilities of Babies.* London: University of London Press.
Hagbarth, K. E., Eklund, G. (1968) 'The effects of muscle vibration in spasticity, rigidity and cerebellar disorders.' *Journal of Neurology, Neurosurgery and Psychiatry,* **31**, 207-213.
Hagberg, B., Lundberg, A. (1969) 'Dissociated motor development simulating cerebral palsy.' *Neuropädiatrie.* **1**, 187-199.

—— Sanner, G., Steen, M. (1972) 'The dysequilibrium syndrome in cerebral palsy.' *Acta Paediatrica Scandinavica*, **61**, Supplement 226.

Hagberg, G., Hagberg, B., Olow, I. (1976) 'The changing panorama of cerebral palsy in Sweden, 1954-1970. III. The importance of fetal deprivation supply.' *Acta Paediatrica Scandinavica*, **65**, 403-408.

Haidvogl, M. (1979) 'Dissociation of maturation: a distinct syndrome of delayed motor development.' *Developmental Medicine and Child Neurology*, **21**, 52-57.

Hammond, W. A. (1871a) *A Treatise on Diseases of the Nervous System*. New York: Appleton.

—— (1871b) On athetosis'. *Medical Times (New York)* **2**, 747.

Hart, H., Bax, M., Jenkins, S. (1978) 'The value of a developmental history.' *Developmental Medicine and Child Neurology*, **20**, 442-452.

Held, R. (1965) 'Plasticity in sensory-motor systems.' *Scientific American*, **213**, (5), 84-94.

Hellbrügge, T., Pechstein, J. (1968) 'Entwicklunspsychologische Tabellen für das Kindesalter.' *Fortschritte der Medizin*, **86**, 481-484.

—— von Wimpffen, J. H. (1975) *Die ersten 365 Tage im Leben eines Kindes. Die Entwicklung des Saüglings*. Munich: Verlags Union.

Hellebrandt, D. T. (1977) 'Motor learning rediscovered. A study of change.' *Cited by* Payton, O. In: *Scientific Bases for Neurophysiologic Approaches to Therapeutic Exercise*. Philadelphia: Davies. pp. 3-35.

Hochleitner, M. (1968) 'Zerebrale Bewegungsstörungen.' *Mitteilungen der Osterreisch Sanitätsverwaltung*, **69**, 2.

—— (1969) 'Pathologisch Haltungs- und Bewegungsmuster beim zerebralparetischen Saügling.' *Fortschritte der Medizin*, **87**, 1091-1097.

Hunter, J. *Cited by* Beevor, C. E. (1903) *loc. cit.*

Illingworth, R. S. (1960) *The Development of the Infant and Young Child, Normal and Abnormal*. Edinburgh: Livingstone. pp. 260-265.

—— (1962) *An Introduction to Development Assessment in the First Year. Little Club Clinics in Developmental Medicine, No. 3*. London: National Spastics Society.

Ingram, T. T. S. (1954) 'The early manifestations and course of diplegia in childhood.' *Archives of Disease in Childhood*, **30**, 244-250.

—— (1962) 'Clinical significance of the infantile feeding reflex.' *Developmental Medicine and Child Neurology*, **4**, 159-169.

—— (1964) *Paediatric Aspects of Cerebral Palsy*. Edinburgh: Churchill Livingstone

—— (1973) 'Soft Signs'. Developmental Medicine and Child Neurology, **15**, 527-9.

Jackson, J. H. (1958) *Selected Writings*. (Taylor, E. H., Ed.) London: Staples Press, **Vol 2**, 29.

Jones, G. B. (1961) 'Dislocation of the hip in asymmetrical spasticity of the thigh adductors.' *Cerebral Palsy Bulletin*, **3**, 190-191.

Kabat, H. (1952) 'Studies in muscular dysfunction. XV: The role of central facilitation in restoration of motor function in paralysis.' *Archives of Physical Medicine*, **33**, 521-533.

—— (1958) 'Proprioceptive facilitation.' In: Licht, S. (ed.) *Therapeutic Exercises*. Baltimore: Waverley Press, **Vol. 3**, Ch. 12.

—— (1959) 'Athetosis: neuromuscular dysfunction and treatment.' *Archives of Physical Medicine*, **40**, 285-292.

Köng, E. (1962) 'Behandlungsresultate bei Früh- und Spätfallen.' *Padiatrische Fortbildung, Praxis*, **1**, 37-38.

—— (1965) Frühdiagnose und Frühbehandlung zerebraler Bewegungsstörungen ("Lähmungen") mit Demonstration von Behandlungsresultaten.' *Praxi*, **54**, 1280-1284.

—— (1966) 'Very early treatment of cerebral palsy.' *Developmental Medicine and Child Neurology*, **8**, 198-202.

Kravitz, H., Goldenberg, D., Neyhus, A. (1978) 'Tactual exploration by normal infants.' *Developmental Medicine and Child Neurology*, **20**, 720-726.

Lesigang, C. (1973) 'Grundsätzliches zur Entwicklungsdiagnostik.' Mitteilungen *Osterreich Sanitatsverwaltung*, **2**.

—— (1976) 'Normalweichedde Motorik im 1 Lebensjahr.' *Diagnostik*, **9**, 538-541.

—— Schwägerl, W. (1974) 'Entwicklungsneurologischer Befunde und Hüftbefund im Säuglingsalter.' *Pädiatrie und Pädologie*, **9**, 344-351.

Lesny, I. (1960) 'The hypotonic forms of cerebral palsy. An analysis of 41 cases and an attempt to explain their origin.' *Cerebral Palsy Bulletin*, **2**, 159-166.

The Little Club (1959) 'Memorandum on terminology and classification of "Cerebral Palsy".' *Cerebral Palsy Bulletin*, **1**, (5), 27-35.

91

Luria, A. R. (1961) *The Role of Speech in the Regulation of Normal and Abnormal Behaviour.* Oxford: Pergamon.

McGraw, M. B. (1963) *The Neuromuscular Maturation of the Human Infant.* New York: Hafner.

Mac Keith, R. C. (1964) 'The primary walking response and its facilitation by passive extension of the head,' *Acta Paediatrica Latina,* **17,** 710.

Magnus, R. (1924) *Körperstellung.* Berlin: Springer. p. 75.

—— (1926) 'Some results of studies of the physiology of posture.' *Lancet,* **2,** 531-535, 585.

Magoun, H. W., Rhines, R. (1946) 'Inhibitory mechanisms in bulbar reticular formation.' *Journal of Neurophysiology,* **9,** 165-171.

—— —— (1948) *Spasticity, the Stretch Reflex and the Extrapyramidal Systems.* Springfield, Illinois: C. C. Thomas.

Manning, J. (1972) 'Facilitation of movement: the Bobath approach.' *Physiotherapy,* **58,** 403-408.

Milani-Comparetti, A. (1964) 'Cerebral palsy in the framework of modern neurophysiology.' *Paper presented at the 4th International Study Group on Child Neurology and Cerebral Palsy, Oxford.*

—— (1965) 'Spasticity versus patterned postural and motor behaviour of spastics.' *Europa Medicophisica,* **1,** (3).

—— Gidoni, E. A. (1967) 'Pattern analysis of motor development and its disorders. *Developmental Medicine and Child Neurology,* **9,** 625-630.

Paine, R. S. (1960) 'Neurological examination of infants and children.' *Pediatric Clinics of North America,* **7,** 471-510.

—— (1964) 'The evolution of infantile postural reflexes in the presence of chronic brain syndromes.' *Developmental Medicine and Child Neurology,* **6,** 345-361.

—— Oppé, T. E. (1966) *Neurological Examination of Children. Clinics in Developmental Medicine, Nos. 20/21.* London: S.I.M.P. with Heinemann; Philadelphia: Lippincott.

Peiper, A. (1961) *Die Eigenart der kindlichen Hirntätigkeit.* Leipzig: Thieme. pp. 155-294.

Perlstein, M. A. (1954) 'Infantile spastic hemiplegia: incidence.' *Pediatrics,* **14,** 436-441.

Polani, P. E. (1959) 'The natural history of choreoathetoid cerebral palsy.' *Guy's Hospital Reports,* **108,** 32-45.

Pollock, G. A. (1955) *The Place of Orthopaedic Surgery in the Treatment of Cerebral Palsy.* London: British Council for the Welfare of Spastics.

Pollock, L. J., Davis, L. (1927) 'Studies in decerebration: integrated reflexes of brain stem.' *Archives of Neurology and Psychiatry,* **17,** 18-23.

Prechtl, H. F. R. (1953) 'Uber die Kopplung von Säugen and Greifen beim Säughling', *Naturwissenschaften,* **40,** 347.

—— (1965) 'Prognostic value of neurological signs in the newborn infant.' *Proceedings of the Royal Society of Medicine,* **58,** 3-4.

—— (1977) *The Neurological Examination of the Full-Term Newborn Infant, 2nd edn. Clinics in Developmental Medicine, No. 63.* London: S.I.M.P. with Heinemann; Philadelphia: Lippincott.

—— Beintema, D. (1964) *The Neurological Examination of the Full-Term Newborn Infant. Little Club Clinics in Developmental Medicine, No. 12.* London: S.I.M.P. with Heinemann; Philadelphia: Lippincott.

Rademaker, G. C. J. (1931) *Das Stehen.* Berlin: Springer.

—— (1935) *Réactions Labyrinthiques et Equilibre.* Paris: Masson.

Riddoch, G., Buzzard, E. F. (1921) 'Reflex movements and postural reactions in quadriplegia and hemiplegia with special reference to those of the upper limb.' *Brain,* **44,** 397-489.

Ritchie-Russell, W. R. (1958) 'The Physiology of memory.' *Proceedings of the Royal Society of Medicine,* **51,** 9.

Robson, R. (1970) 'Shuffling, hitching, scooting and sliding: some observations in 30 otherwise normal children.' *Developmental Medicine and Child Neurology,* **12,** 608-617.

—— Mac Keith, R. C. (1971) 'Shufflers with spastic displegic cerebral palsy: a confusing clinical picture.' *Developmental Medicine and Child Neurology,* **13,** 651-659.

Rood, M. (1956) 'Neurophysiological mechanism utilised in the treatment of neuromuscular dysfunction.' *American Journal of Occupational Therapy,* **10,** 220-225.

—— (1962) 'The use of sensory receptors to activate, facilitate and inhibit motor responses, automatic and somatic, in developmental sequence.' In' Sattely, G. C. (ed). *Approaches to Treatment of Patients with Neuromuscular Dysfunction,* 26-37. Dubuque, Iowa: William C. Brown.

Rosenbloom, L. (1971) 'The contribution of motor behaviour to child development.' *Physiotherapy,* **57,** 159-162.

—— (1975) 'The consequences of impaired movement—an hypothesis and review.' In: Holt, K. S. (Ed.)

Movement and Child Development, Clinics in Developmental Medicine, No. 55. London: S.I.M.P. with Heinemann; Philadelphia: Lippincott.

Rushworth, G. (1960) 'Spasticity and rigidity. An experimental study and review.' *Journal of Neurology, Neurosurgery and Psychiatry,* **23,** 99-118.

—— (1961) 'On postural and righting reflexes'. *Cerebral Palsy Bulletin,* **3,** 535-543.

Samilson, R. L. (1975) *Orthopaedic Aspects of Cerebral Palsy. Clinics in Developmental Medicine, Nos. 52/53.* London: S.I.M.P. with Heinemann; Philadelphia: Lippincott.

Sanner, G. (1971) 'Non-progressive ataxic syndromes in childhood.' Paper presented at the seventh meeting of the Scandinavian Group of Paediatric Neurology, May 20—21, Tonsberg, Norway.

Schaltenbrand, G. (1925) 'Normale Bewegungs-und Lägereaktionen bei Kindern.' *Deutsche Zeischrift für Nervenheilkunde,* **87,** 23-59.

—— (1926) 'Uber die Entwicklung des menschlichen Aufstehens und dessen Störungen bei verscheidenen Nervenkrankheiten.' *Deutsche Zeitschrift für Nervenheilkunde,* **89,** 82-90.

—— (1927) 'The development of human motility and motor disturbances.' *Bulletin of the New York Academy of Medicine,* **3,** 534-536.

Semans, S. (1967) 'The Bobath concept in treatment of neurological disorders. A neuro-developmental treatment.' *American Journal of Physical Therapy,* **46,** 732-788.

Sharrard, W. J. W. (1961) 'Danger of dislocation of the hip in asymmetrical spasticity of the thigh adductors.' *Cerebral Palsy Bulletin,* **3,** 72-73.

Sheridan, M. D. (1968) *The Developmental Progress of Infants and Young Children. 2nd edn.* London: H.M.S.O.

—— (1973) *Children's Developmental Progress from Birth to Five Years. The STYCAR Sequences.* Windsor: N.F.E.R.

Sherrington, C. S. (1913) 'Reflex inhibition as a factor in the co-ordination of movements and postures.' *Quarterly Journal of Experimental Physiology,* **6,** 251-310.

—— (1934) 'Reflex inhibition as a factor in co-ordination of muscular acts.' *Revista de la Sociedad Argentina de Biologia,* Supplement 10, 510-513.

—— (1947) *The Integrative Action of the Nervous System.* Cambridge: C.U.P.

Skatvedt, M. (1961) 'Early treatment of hemiplegia.' In: *Hemiplegic Cerebral Palsy in Children and Adults. Little Club Clinics in Developmental Medicine, No. 4.* London: National Spastics Society with Heinemann Medical.

Snell, E. E. (1976) In: Cruickshank, W. M. (Ed.) *Cerebral Palsy: A Developmental Disability.* Syracuse, N.Y.: Syracuse University Press. p. 39.

Tardieu, G. (1961) 'Danger of dislocation of the hip in asymmetrical spasticity of the thigh adductors.' *Cerebral Palsy Bulletin,* **3,** 71.

Tizard, J. (1961) Observations on the early manifestations of infantile hemiplegia.' In: *Hemiplegic Cerebral Palsy in Children and Adults. Little Club Clinics in Developmental Medicine, No. 4.* London: National Spastics Society with Heinemann Medical.

Touwen, B. C. L. (1976) *Neurological Development in Infancy. Clinics in Developmental Medicine, No. 58.* London: S.I.M.P. with Heinemann; Philadelphia: Lippincott.

—— Prechtl, H. F. R. (1970) *The Neurological Examination of the Child with Minor Nervous Dysfunction. Clinics in Developmental Medicine, No. 38.* London: S.I.M.P. with Heinemann; Philadelphia: Lippincott.

Tower, S. S. (1935) 'Dissociation of cortical excitation, from cortical inhibition by pyramidal section, and the syndrome of that lesion in the cat.' *Brain,* **58,** 238-255.

—— (1940) 'Pyramidal lesion in the monkey.' *Brain,* **63,** 36-90.

Treml, H. (1975) 'Die motorische Entwicklung des hemiplegischen Kindes und therapeutische Massnahmen zur Beeinflussung des pathologischen Bildes.' In: *Spezielle Probleme des hemiplegischen Kindes.* Dusseldorf: Bundesverband für spastisch Gelahmte.

Twitchell, T. E. J. (1954) 'Sensory factors in purposive movements.' *Journal of Neurophysiology,* **17,** 239-252.

Uexkuell, J. van (1904) 'Studien über den Tonus, II: Die Bewegungen der Schlangensterne.' *Zeitschrift für Biologie,* **46,** 1-37.

—— (1905) 'Studien über den Tonus, III: Die Blutegel.' *Zeitschrift für Biologie,* **46,** 372-402.

Vojta, V. (1974) *Die cerebralen Bewegungsstörungen in Säuglingsalter.* Stuttgart: Enke.

Vassella, F., Karlsson, B. (1962) 'Asymmetric tonic neck reflex. A review of the literature and a study of its presence in the neonatal period.' *Developmental Medicine and Child Neurology,* **4,** 363-369.

Walshe, F. M. R. (1921) 'On disorders of movement resulting from loss of postural tone with special reference to cerebellar ataxy.' *Brain,* **44,** 539-556.

—— (1923) 'On certain tonic or postural reflexes in adult hemiplegia, with special reference to associated and so-called associated movements.' *Brain,* **46,** 2-23.

—— (1948) *Critical Studies in Neurology.* Edinburgh: Livingstone.

Wasz-Höckert, O., Lind, J., Vuorenkoski, V., Partanen, T., Valanne, E. (1968) *The Infant Cry. A Spectrographic and Auditory Analysis. Clinics in Developmental Medicine, No. 29.* London: S.I.M.P. with Heinemann; Philadelphia: Lippincott.

Weisz, S. (1938) 'Studies in equilibrium reaction.' *Journal of Nervous and Mental Diseases,* **88,** 150-162.

Wilson, S. A. K. (1920) 'On decerebrate rigidity in man and the occurrence of tonic fits.' *Brain,* **43,** 220-268.

—— (1925) 'The Croonian Lectures on some disorders of motility and muscle tone with special reference to the corpus striatum.' *Lancet,* **2,** 169-178.

—— Walshe, F. M. R. (1914/15) 'The phenomenon of tonic innervation and its relation to motor apraxia.' *Brain,* **37,** 199-246.

Zador, J. (1938) *Les Reactions d'Equilibre chez l'Homme.* Paris: Masson.

Zappella, M. (1964) 'Postural Reactions in 100 children with cerebral palsy and mental handicap.' *Developmental Medicine and Child Neurology,* **6,** 475-484.

INDEX

Note: Due to the close proximity of illustrations to the relevant text, no page numbers for illustrations have been included. *f* indicates footnote.

Extensor pattern of palsy—*cont.*
   tonus 38
      1-10 months 19
      hypertonus, maximal 68
Exteroceptors initiation of motor response 78, 83

F

Facilitation principle, of treatment 77, 84
   effect 86
Finger-nose test 58
Fleeting localised contractions, in athetoid palsy
   62
Flexion
   contractures, hip and knee 23
   lower extremities, competition with exten-
     sion 84
   neonatal 11
Flexor
   deformities, of athetoid palsy 65
   hypertonus 36, 70
   withdrawal reflex 79
Floppy infant
   differential diagnosis 57
   myotatic responses, variability 29
   tests 72

G

Galant reaction 15
   1-10 months 20
Gamma activity, evoked 87
   role in spasticity 28, 29
Grasp response, association with sucking reflex
   3
   neonatal 12
   of the spastic diplegic 53
   relation to speech and articulation 3*f*

H

Habit patterns, neurological 78
Handling, limit of tolerance 85
Hands, neonatal, normal motor co-ordination 14
Head control
   1-10 months 20
   in righting reactions 7
   in spastic quadriplegia 47
   Moro reflex test 13
Head-raising, symmetrical tonic neck reflex 40
Head-turning, asymmetrical tonic neck reflex 38
Hemiplegia, definition 45
   double 45
   early signs 75
   spastic 54-56
Higher reactions, facilitation 86
Hip
   dislocation 14
     athetoid palsy 63, 65
     spastic diplegia 53
     spastic quadriplegia 50
   extension, normal 14
Hypertonus
   plastic 28, 30
   rotatory therapy 6
Hypotonic palsy. *See* Floppy infant

I

Infants, newborn, normal motor co-ordination 11
Ingram's ataxic diplegia 61, 72
Inhibition, spinal animal 80
Inhibitory control, formation 85
Intact animal 81
Interpretation of handicap, role in treatment 82
Involuntary movement, types, in athetoid palsy 61

K

Key points, of inhibitory control 85
Kicking pattern 14, 20
Kneeling position, symmetrical tonic neck reflex
   40
Kyphoscoliosis, athetoid palsy 65
Kyphosis, compensatory 49

L

Labyrinthine reflex, tonic 34-38
   righting reaction 8
     neonatal 14
Landau reaction 21, 24
Legs, neonatal, normal motor co-ordination 14
Lower extremities, competing patterns 84
Lumbar lordosis, compensatory 52

M

Magnus, on rule of shunting 83
Maturation, brain, correlation with motor co-
   ordination 4
   neurological, 'three-monthly period' 27
Midbrain (thalamic) animal 80
Mobile spasms, of athetoid palsy 62
Moro reflex 13
   athetoid palsy 64
   disappearance 23
   spastic diplegia 52
Mother-child relationship, development 2
   observation, in assessment 67
Motor
   co-ordination, correlation with brain matu-
     ration 4
     normal 11-25
   development, in ataxic children 58
   function, integration 79
   pattern, sparsity, in the cerebral palsied child
     31
Muscles
   control of CNS 83
   co-ordination 5
     abnormal patterns 32
   reciprocal innervation 5
Myotatic responses 29

N

Neck
   asymmetric tonic neck reflex 12, 38, 73
   righting reaction 8
     neonatal 14
   symmetrical tonic neck reflex 40
Neonates, motor co-ordination, normal 11
Neurophysiology 77